The Weighing Game
& How To Win It
WITHOUT GETTING SICK OR GOING BROKE

The Weighing Game & How To Win It

WITHOUT GETTING SICK OR GOING BROKE

by Ottone and Dolores Riccio

Book Design by James Doddy

Rodale Press, Inc., Book Division, Emmaus, Pa. 18049

International Standard Book
Number 0-87857-081-0
Library of Congress Catalog '
Number 73-21132
Copyright © 1974 by Rodale Press

Printed in the United States of America
Printed on recycled paper

First Printing   May 1974
PB-296

Riccio, Dolores, 1931-
    Weighing game and how to win it.

    1. Reducing diets.   I. Riccio, Ottone,
1921-   joint author.   II. Title.
RM222.2.R48   613.2'5   73-21132
ISBN 0-87857-081-0

Contents

1807890

Page

An Introduction to "The Game" **1**

Chapter **1** **Deciding on the Name of the Game** . . . **6**
"An Inch to the Pinch"
Willpower Is Not Enough (but a Little
Won't Power Helps!)
Poor Little Rich Kids and How They
Get Fat
It's a Big Problem!
Big Problems Need Big Answers

Chapter **2** **Learning the Rules** **15**
Shaving Rabbits, and Other Interesting
Experiments
Just Like Mother Used To Make
Throwing a Monkey Wrench into the
Metabolism
"But I Eat Like a Bird!"

Chapter **3** **Has Heredity Put You behind the
Eight Ball?** **24**
A Few Facts and Figures about Figures
and Fat
Twiggy, Sophia, and Liz
Fat Cells Are Stranger Than Fiction
Riding on a Vicious Cycle
Improving Your Mathematical Skills

Chapter **4** **You're Out!—You're Not Playing the Game** **36**
Obesity and Its Evil Companions
The View from the Family Album
Alexander Bell, the Wright Brothers,
    et al

Chapter **5** **Think Thin and Win** **45**
"I'm in the Mood for Food"
"I Ate It Because It Was There"
"Mirror, Mirror on the Wall . . ."
"Eat Fast, or You'll Fast"

Chapter **6** **"The Cards Are Stacked against Me!"** **64**
"A Barrel of Laughs . . ."
A Rousing Cheer for Change

Chapter **7** **Play To Block "Future Fat"** **74**
Bootleg Beefburgers, Anyone?
Future Fat

Chapter **8** **If You're Not Winning, Switch Courts** **84**
"But I Made It Just for You!"
"Nothin' Says Lovin' Like Something
    from the Oven" and Other
    Misconceptions
Getting It All Together

Chapter **9** **Solitaire—Don't Cheat the Dealer** **95**
On Leading a Life of Diet Desperation

Chapter **10** **The Public Is the Pawn** **104**
The Not-So-Good Old Days
Perspectives—Yesterday, Today, and
    Tomorrow

Chapter **11** **Fat Chance** **112**

"Make Mine Vanilla"
"Why Do You Go On Straining Your
Willpower?"
How To Be the Toast of the "Talk
Shows"
The Fast Way
The Slow Way
The Revolutionary Way

Chapter **12** **The Diet Business—Rakes in the
Chips** **146**

God Sends Meat and the Devil Sends
Preservatives
Zen in the Art of Dieting
"Don't Call Me, I'll Call You"
Biofeedback Is Better Than No Feed
at All

Chapter **13** **Bet Your Life on a Rainbow Pill!** **161**

"Crashing" to Reality with Diet Drugs
The Right To Ask Questions—and To
Get Answers
The Pep-Pill Generation
Diet Drugs: the Loser's Game

Chapter **14** **"Go for Broke"—Buy Expensive
Reducing Equipment** **197**

Sauna Treatments Are "Hot Stuff"
Shake, Rattle, and Roll Your Way to a
New Figure
"How I Spent My Summer Vacation"
The Massage Is the Message
"Tenting Tonight on the Old Camp
Ground"
Trends in Getting Trim

Page

Chapter **15** **Exercise Has the Inside Track** **230**
Neat Exercises for Small Spaces
Big Exercises for Wide, Open Spaces
Graceful Exercises for Mirrored Rooms
Rolling through Those Rolling Hills
Keep Moving—and You'll Keep Young

Chapter **16** **It's a Whole New Game** **243**
Survival in the Supermarket
How To Say "Good Morning"—and
Mean It!
High-Test Fuel for a First Class Engine
How To Avoid That "Empty Feeling"
More Bounce to the Ounce
Divide and Conquer
Munching to Your Heart's Content
The Lively Way of Life

Chapter **17** **The Winner Loses—the Loser Wins** . . . **267**
Treat Yourself Royally
Party It Up
Husband Keeping
Burning Your Bridges
Life without an Adding Machine
"It's Not Nice To Fool Mother Nature"
Welcome to a New World

Index **276**

An Introduction to "The Game"

Ever since some enterprising snake-oil merchandiser tucked the heads of tapeworms into capsules and sold them as reducing pills, those who would like to be a little (or a lot) thinner have been the unwitting victims of the entrepreneurs of the Body Beautiful.

With trusting innocence, people have bathed in reducing salts, nibbled reducing "candy," shaken themselves silly on vibrating tables, swallowed any number of mystery pills, and confined their natural appetites to weird restrictive diets, some of which contain no food at all. Yielding their bodies to what might have been called "torture" in another, more honest age, they've sweated in steam rooms where the temperature reaches 200 degrees, swathed their limbs in tightly-wound "mummy" bandages, and consented to wear heavily weighted garments on their hips and thighs while they "relaxed" around the house. In extreme cases, they've even allowed their bodies to be cut open in order to remove that offending portion of the intestine which insists upon absorbing nutrition from the food they ate. In short, there is no discomfort, inconvenience, or danger to which the public is not willing to submit in the unending quest for the elusive miracle, a shapely, physically-fit body.

Strangely enough, the one approach they have always been reluctant to adopt is a moderate and balanced one, although they enthusiastically embrace extreme measures like starvation, drugs, hypnotism, and the use of mysterious machines in their search.

Even otherwise sober and sensible adults, who wouldn't dream of writing checks on a non-existent bank balance, believe in that something-for-nothing fairy tale whereby a person falls asleep at night as his usual pudgy and amuscular self—and wakes the next morning marvellously changed into the slim and svelte person of his dreams, ready to marry the prince or princess and live happily ever after. Advertising copy writers are well aware of the public's weakness for certain key words, like "magic," "easy," "effortless," "revolutionary," and "while you sleep."

After the drugs, the pounding, wrapping, stewing, steaming, and two weeks of subsisting wholly on grapefruit, cottage cheese, and chemical, low-cal colas, does anyone actually *lose* anything? YES! Some people lose inches from waist and hips for a few hours. Some lose pounds for a few days. Some lose their tempers and all but their most devoted friends. The public loses millions of dollars each year. But, worse than that, some lose good health, and even life itself in pursuit of "the body beautiful."

It doesn't have to be that grim, however, every time you reduce your bank account in order to reduce your figure. You can spend lots of money on remedies that won't hurt you at all—and won't do you very much good either! The *Wall Street Journal* reports an estimated sale of $100 million a year on "effortless" exercise equipment to shock, shake, rattle, and roll you into the American Ideal. You can join a club for moral support and saccharine-loaded recipes, subscribe to a telephone service for daily nagging from an anonymous friend who inquires into your eating habits, or pray your weight away with the aid of an instructive text. You can follow diets proposed by persons from all walks of life, from television stars to plastic surgeons, from mystic readers to medicine men of all persuasions.

Then there are the "reducing aids" sold over the counter of your local drug store or through the mails, with advertisements that read like *True Confessions:* "I lost my matronly look when I lost 70 pounds," "These women lost 509 pounds and found work, love, success, beauty, excitement, and even jealousy." Unfortunately, none of these "aids" actually works unless you also follow the accompanying *diet* secreted inside the gaily-colored package with the picture of a lithe model in a brief bikini.

The postal department has a regular game of bringing charges for false advertising against the makers of reducing aids sold through the mails. Whereupon the company disbands, leaves town, and starts a new life in a new location with another seductive product name. We have no law against a fresh start in this land of opportunity!

With obesity as a health problem assuming the proportions of a national epidemic, perhaps the time has come for a return to common sense, that uncommon quality, and an unsparing evaluation of the hoaxes and hucksters of the fleece-the-fat game. It's time, too, to take an honest look at ourselves (preferably in the mirror), at our families and our "rich" society. Half the people we know are on a diet, many claim they are "too busy" to exercise, and almost everyone is looking for a "short cut" to physical fitness. (Regrettably, some persist in looking for it in the refrigerator at midnight!)

In order to appraise ourselves and those we love in terms of physical fitness, it's important to sort through a great amount of published material on obesity and discover what the term really means. Is it the word that ought to be used in describing your own pleasingly plump figure? Why is the prognosis so discouraging for obesity? The desperate fatties of the world have provided an almost unlimited supply of experimental subjects for every possible "cure" of this number-one health problem, with a depressing lack of success. In this book we propose some life-plan alternatives, with an emphasis on feeling good as well as looking good, as an antidote for the general atmosphere of quackery and short-term miracle working that surrounds the dieter in our time.

The subject of exercise, too, needs to be analyzed and put into proper perspective. Exercise doesn't have to be expensive, lonely, or boring, and we believe that it is just as important as many of the other activities to which most people are now donating their valuable time. We suggest, also, that exercise is a vital component of any reducing program.

There is (and always has been) a perfectly natural, sensible, well-balanced, healthy, and inexpensive way to restore physical fitness. It does not require the use of slimming belts, electric muscle machines, fudge-flavored diet cookies, a portable sauna, or a club house. All it does require is a little time, a little care and thoughtful planning in regard to what one eats and how one exercises—the kind of care we would expect to give any valuable possession. When a new car is purchased, people know it's not enough to just polish the chrome and step on the gas pedal. They know that the needs of the engine must be considered. And so it is with the even more intricate and precious body. It can't be turned in every two or three years for a new model. Happily, though, the body was not designed for early obsolescence, and, if proper care is taken, it will last for a long and healthy lifetime.

And so, like Alice stepping through the looking-glass into Wonderland, let's wrap ourselves up in sauna towels, take our pocket calorie counters in hand, and wander into the wild and wacky world of The Weighing Game . . .

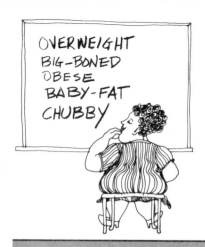

Deciding on the Name of the Game

"The heaviest human on record weighed 1,069 pounds and was buried in a piano case," according to *The Guinness Book of World Records*—and this, without doubt, was a clear-cut case of obesity! But the line between obesity and mere overweight (a much more socially acceptable term) is not always so easily defined. Many persons who optimistically think of themselves as "a little bit heavy" are quick to diagnose a case of genuine obesity in someone else.

Obese people are all overweight, but not all overweight people are obese. Dr. George A. Bray makes this distinction writing in the *American Journal of Clinical Nutrition:* obesity exists when fat (the stores of fatty tissue beneath the skin) makes up a greater than normal fraction of the total body weight; overweight, on the other hand, applies chiefly to how much heavier you are than the recommended weight for your age, sex, and body frame, according to the standard weight charts. Technically, you are overweight if you weigh 116 pounds, when the chart says you should weigh 112.

People consulting such a chart have no choice about listing their sex and something soothingly called their "age range," but, when it comes to body frame, almost all overweight people cheerfully claim a large frame. "I'm big-boned, don't you think, doctor?" many a chubby lady has been heard to ask pleadingly, when the chips were down (and her weight was up), deliberately ignoring her narrow shoulders and her dainty wrists.

Of all the hoaxes which will be described in this book, the most damaging may very well be *self*-hoaxing, the little strategies people use to delude themselves about their own bodies.

But even with the best of intentions, trying to determine your weight problem by consulting weight charts can be confusing. You have to choose among "average" weight charts, "ideal" weight charts, charts prepared by insurance companies and charts prepared by government agencies, and each of these is revised from time to time. Moreover, many experts hold that the charts available to the layman do not include sufficient data on differing body types to enable him to judge his own correctly. There is also evidence that one person's "ideal" weight is another person's fat tummy.

That's why, no matter how honestly you think you have assessed your mini- or maxi-bone structure, it is a good idea to try one or two of the more pragmatic "home tests" for obesity in the privacy of your own bedroom. (Remember—you don't have to reveal the results to a soul!)

"An Inch to the Pinch"

Two simple tests which indicate whether one is "overly-larded" were suggested by Lawrence Galton, a science writer, in an article in the *New York Times Magazine.* A layer of fat one-fourth to one-half of an inch thick under the skin is normal, according to **Mr.** Galton, but if, when you take "a deep pinch of flesh on the side of the body just over the lower ribs" and "the spread between thumb and index finger exceeds an inch, there's too much fat." Too much fat, of course, is the key to obesity.

The same test may be applied to the fleshy underside of the arm between the elbow and the shoulder.

The second test recommended by Mr. Galton is "to lie flat and place a twelve-inch ruler on your abdomen, with one end between the flare of your ribs. If the ruler stays flat, congratulations; if it points ceiling-ward, you're fat."

Professional methods of determining the degree of obesity are much more elaborate (not to mention more expensive). They range from the external methods— the development of skinfold measurements and measuring tapes, combined with accurate weighing of the individual and determination of body type—all the way to internal measurement methods—estimating the number of "fat cells", and using these data to calculate the total amount of fat.

However, if you can determine your own weight problem objectively and learn to deal with it effectively, you might avoid the complicated medical regimens that are imposed on the dangerously obese. No need to wait for your yearly medical exam to find out that you ought to change your eating and exercise habits. Many persons have arrived at that conclusion by simply looking in the mirror and honestly observing what is revealed there.

Although the diagnosis of obesity can be as easy as taking a good, long look at a candid beach photograph (determined souls will tape the most unflattering one to the refrigerator!), discovering the causes of and the cure for obesity is not always so easy. Possible, yes—but not easy.

"Willpower" Is Not Enough (but a Little Won't Power Helps!)

Not so long ago, authorities on obesity were proclaiming the theory that overweight is solely the result of overeating. Willful overeating. Gluttony. There was an elementary equation involved, much like balancing a checkbook: if a person takes in more food energy, in the form of calories, than he expends in activity, the unused energy will be stored in the body as fat. Losing weight, therefore, is just a matter of reversing the process—taking in *less* food energy than is expended.

This reversal of the process of "deposit" and "withdrawal" was named a "reducing diet"—a person stayed on such a diet until he reached his ideal weight.

This act of self-denial required an elusive quality known as "will power."

As a result of this line of thinking, fat people who failed to become thin were looked upon as "weak-willed," hardly able to pass a bakery without stopping in to sample the forbidden fruit-cakes. Thus did the obese become the guilt-ridden, misunderstood, and oppressed folk of society.

First of all, let's affirm that this "bank account" theory is basically true, but it is *not the whole story*. Overeating for a long period of time usually causes overweight (especially if one is eating the wrong kinds of food), but there is increasing evidence that many other factors can contribute to the condition of obesity, aside from caloric imbalance.

For example, researchers have learned that some obese persons actually do not eat any more than non-obese persons. They may even eat *less*. (And the worst of it is, no one believes that the chubby girl has been subsisting on an occasional lettuce sandwich while her Audrey Hepburn-type friend has gorged herself on hot fudge sundaes without guilt and without gaining a gram.) Many obese individuals lose weight very slowly and with great difficulty even under strict supervision and calorie control within the confines of a hospital.

Dr. Felix Heald of the Children's Hospital in Washington, D.C., stated, in the *Journal of the American Medical Association,* "For too long, we have considered obesity primarily a gourmet-determined syndrome and have attempted to treat it as such. Our lack of success in such an approach probably is a testimonial to our lack of knowledge about the multi-determined etiology of obesity."

This new light shed on the problem of obesity is to be welcomed, but with it come two new dangers. The first is the aura of hopelessness that pervades so much of the current professional medical literature on obesity. From the era of "all you need is a little will power" we have come full circle to the era of "the poor devil can't help himself." This gives rise to the second danger: the variety of available excuses the obese person can find for doing nothing about his problem, knowing that his family history and psychological problems may be contributing to it.

We are learning that solutions may not be as fast and simple as the once-popular 7-day miracle diets (the miracle being that one can endure seven days on something like bananas and skim milk), but there *are* solutions—that's the important thing.

The application of "Won't power" can begin with the vow, "I won't be hopeless. And I won't be helpless either."

Poor Little Rich Kids and How They Get Fat

In underdeveloped areas of the world, where food is usually scarce—a coarse, repetitive, unrefined fare—and everyone works hard for it, obesity is virtually non-existent. In fact, where the fear of starvation exists, the few women who manage to be plump are generally considered the most beautiful.

In a country as rich as America, where food is abundant to large masses of the population, obesity is a major problem. Americans must learn to cope with abundance and variety—and to construct a sensible diet out of the glittering array of foods in the neighbor-hood supermarket.

The supermarket managers pretend to help by stocking their shelves with "diet foods" for those fat-and-guilty shoppers who have already gained too much weight from indulging in the cakes, cookies, candies, frozen creamed casseroles, and potato chips sold on the other aisles of the store. Just what kind of a diet these "diet foods" provide remains to be seen, but one thing is certain: this is a part of the game in which only the supermarket is the winner.

It's a Big Problem!

That people are interested and even anxious to learn all they can about obesity is obvious from the voluminous data flowing from the popular press, radio, and television. This isn't surprising when you realize that 50 percent of the people in America are over-weight. But sad to say, some of the "advice" being of-fered by the media is beyond the realm of common sense.

For example, Dr. Irwin M. Stillman's book, *The Doctor's Quick Weight Loss Diet,* advises: *"Guard Against Food and Diet 'Myths' That Lead You Astray.* Many people have the craziest notions about what constitutes 'healthful eating.' Often the food myths have been fostered by constant, costly propaganda by special interests or misguided 'food and nutrition ex-perts' . . . Even for the overweight youngster, a small ball of ice cream and nothing else would be a more healthful breakfast since it would total fewer calories than those 'heaping hot breakfast' specialties."

And so, off through the February snows to school for the ice cream-nourished youngster?

Truly, as Dr. Stillman points out, it's not necessary to consume a breakfast of home fries and pancakes while attempting to lose weight. But mothers somewhere are probably taking Dr. Stillman seriously and, to the question, "What's for breakfast?", they reply, "How about half a scoop of tutti-frutti?"

Big Problems Need Big Answers

Is the obese person a compulsive eater, a food addict? Does his home environment cause or encourage him to eat more than he needs? Is he less active than he should be? Is the appetite-regulating mechanism in his brain functioning improperly? Does he have a behavioral problem or a metabolic one? Has he inherited his tendency toward obesity? Diagnosis is difficult because obesity may be due to any one of these factors or to any combination of them.

But there are means by which obesity can be accurately diagnosed; there are available data on the roles of the appetite-regulating mechanism, hereditary influences, impairment of physical functions, and other physical disorders directly related to obesity. We are beginning, too, to understand the psychological motivations toward obesity.

Knowledge is the key to uncovering the truth about all the misinformation which has been deluging the luckless 50 percent of the population who have chubby tendencies. How much will it profit you to lose five pounds in two days on the Cottage Cheese Blitz Diet? Will an electric exercise machine really harden that flab into muscle with no effort at all on your part? Is there a magic pill you can take?

For answers to these and other fascinating questions, let's move on to the next episode in the perils of the roly-poly dieter.

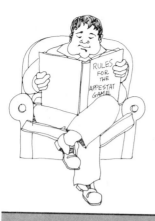

Learning the Rules

Perhaps you've always believed that the little voice whispering in your ear at meal times—the one that tells you you're still hungry and would like a second helping of devil's food cake—must be the devil's own. Maybe you also imagine that a person who says, "No, thanks—I'll just have coffee," is fortunate enough to have a guardian angel whispering in *his* ear. There is, however, a less metaphysical explanation, and it's called the appestat.

The appestat mechanism is believed to be a cluster of cells located in the hypothalamus, a gland tucked deep in the midbrain. It seems to regulate an individual's appetite by signaling when he should start eating to get necessary nourishment, and when he should stop because his body has had enough. That is, when it's working correctly.

You probably know people whose weight never varies, even during times when they are inactive, because their appetites adjust to whatever amount of exercise they perform in the course of their daily lives. They rarely lose a pound, or gain one. No succulent tidbit, no matter how fond they are of it, can tempt them when they're not ready to eat. Such a person has even been known to put his fork down in the middle of a meal and just quit eating, because he no longer feels hungry. No cleaning up his plate "like a good boy." No forcing down just one more spoonful because it's "my favorite." No worry that "it's a shame to waste it while people are starving." He simply knows when he's had enough and stops eating. This individual is among the most envied in America today! He is the fortunate owner of a perfectly functioning appestat.

But, as Harvard nutrition expert, Dr. Jean Mayer, has said, whimsically, "When you have any mechanism, it is likely to obey one of my favorite natural laws—Murphy's Law—which can be stated succinctly as: 'If anything can go wrong, it will.'" Evidently, the appestat in humans is a mechanism which frequently goes wrong—and it only has to go a little wrong to result in a lot of excess poundage.

If one were to eat just one ounce a day more than the body needs, during a year's time, then, in theory, one would have increased his weight by 23 pounds. To put it another way, just 100 calories a day too much will result in a ten pound gain per year. One hundred calories is just a "little snack" to many people—a can of beer in the afternoon, or a couple of cookies before bed—that sort of thing!

On the bright side, though, giving up what represents 100 calories is not a great sacrifice. Just doing without the sugar in coffee and tea would deduct about 100 per day for most people. Everything else being equal, that should result in a ten pound loss per year, according to the caloric calculation method of dieting.

Shaving Rabbits, and Other Interesting Experiments

Scientists have demonstrated the presence and operation of some appetite-regulating mechanism in animals in various experiments: they shaved the hair off rabbits, thus increasing energy expenditure through heat loss, and the animals increased their food intake. When the researchers diluted the food of rats by adding non-nutrient materials, the rats automatically ate more.

Animal experiments have demonstrated that the cell cluster in the hypothalamus is divided into two distinct regions. Injury to one of these regions caused the experimental animal to eat continuously and to grow enormous in size. Injury to the other region caused the animal to refuse food even when it was placed in the animal's mouth. The control mechanism's two halves apparently complement each other, one half stimulating or directing the desire to eat and the other signaling the time to suspend food intake. These two halves, together, form the appetite-regulating mechanism.

Without this regulator, animals would die of starvation with food in front of them, or gorge themselves to death, unaware that they should stop eating. Yet, even outside of the lab, animals' appestats seem to operate much more reliably than those of humans. It has been pointed out by Dr. Mayer that animals of normal weight have an instinctive talent for adjusting food consumption to energy expenditure.

Dr. Donald W. Thomas, a research psychologist working with Dr. Mayer, explains, in cases of animal studies, that animals who have received injuries to the appetite control mechanism fail to wait long enough before eating. He says that oversized meals "set the metabolic system on overtime and a larger percentage of the food eaten is turned into stored fat instead of available nutrients." The result is that the body finds itself short of necessary nutrients and sends out a signal to "start eating" sooner than is really necessary.

Light, nourishing meals, then, would tend to have the opposite effect, to right the metabolic rate—which is something to keep in mind when planning diet menus.

Another thing to keep in mind is that animals who remain in their natural environment manage to adjust their appetites to their needs. This indicates that there is something more at work here than purely involuntary physical causes, something about the very condition of human civilization which is acting upon the appestat in a detrimental fashion.

Just Like Mother Used To Make

More needs to be learned about how appetite itself functions, but it is generally accepted that appetite is influenced by how food looks, smells, tastes, its variety, its temperature, by previous food consumption, recent activity, by habit, and by several psychological factors. In other words, coming home after a day spent swimming and sailing, for example, and sniffing the delicious scent of your favorite food in the oven, cooked-just the way your mother used to make it, is bound to give you a whopping big appetite!

The appetite regulating mechanism can also be influenced by any number of other factors, such as measles, a severe cold, a mild concussion, tumors, sleeping sickness, surgery, and, of course, drugs.

The discovery that drugs influence appetite has been a bonanza for many a drug company. However, it is the A.M.A.'s position that any drug safe enough to be sold without a prescription (drug store and mail order "reducing aids" fall into this category) "will have no value for weight-reducing based on its effect on the body metabolism." On the other hand, "any drug which would stimulate metabolism to such an extent that it would cause weight loss is much too dangerous for use without medical supervision." That means an effective drug can only be sold to you with a prescription. But does that remove the danger?

It's fairly common knowledge now that these prescription diet drugs have harmful side-effects. Did you know, though, that the term "side-effects" in itself may be misleading? Our source is the A.M.A. Journal, Dr. Walter Modell: ". . .it would be much more realistic to view these *not as side-effects but as part of the outstanding pharmacological action of the drugs,* with distraction of the abnormal appetite being a *secondary* effect." (The italics are ours.)

"Public knowledge of why people become obese is now about at the kindergarten stage; it has not kept pace with the rapid spread of the valid doctrine that obesity is a health hazard to be avoided," states Dr. Roger Williams in his book, *Nutrition Against Disease*. He supports the "appestat mechanism" theory and points out that the cells that constitute the mechanism are living tissue just like other cells in the body—they have specific functions and they will perform these functions satisfactorily if they are provided with a healthy environment, as long as there isn't anything "inherently or unalterably wrong" with the mechanism. Nutrition, then, which promotes good health in the entire body, can be considered a positive influence on the appestat.

Some researchers imply a close connection between psychological factors and the operation of the appestat. Anxiety or excitement may temporarily eliminate the desire for food, or *may increase it*. A comfortable atmosphere can be conducive to overeating. Boredom or frustration can produce what is known as "the compulsive eater," one who is supposed to eat as an alcoholic drinks, not to reach a pleasant state of relaxation, but to reach a kind of stupor.

Of course, every person has to deal with emotional states ranging from comfort to frustration and anxiety. Life's common experiences make some people compulsive eaters. Most of these people, however, have sufficient motivation to try all manner of new diets and wonder-cures for fatness, and, if this motivation can just be channeled in the direction of responsible advice and sensible regimens, real success is possible.

The inefficient regulation of appetite as a cause for obesity is cited by numerous researchers. To maintain an ideal weight over a period of years requires a precise balance between the food you eat and the activities in which you engage. With this in mind, it really is amazing that many people are able to keep a more or less constant weight, faced as they are with the rich and varied diet available in our country today—all the way from the haute cuisine of exotic ethnic restaurants to a bucket of Kentucky Fried Chicken at a roadside stand.

Throwing a Monkey Wrench into the Metabolism

"Metabolism" denotes the sum of chemical changes in living beings by which food is converted into energy and living tissue.

As we have seen, it is through signals from the appestat to the metabolism that the demon "appetite" is invoked and/or controlled. To the obese, at any rate, it may seem like a demon when they find themselves reaching for seconds in double-fudge cake, but, actually, an appetite is a necessary attribute in keeping us healthy. Once we have it operating for and not against us, appetite can become what is should be— one of the great pleasures in life.

Naturally, it has occurred to scientists that, if the rate of the metabolism can be manipulated (usually, by the use of drugs), the weight of a person can be affected. An increased rate of metabolism results in

faster conversion of food consumed into energy, whereas a slower rate results in more food stored as fat
when things are proceeding in a normal manner.

· One of the drugs used in weight reduction is the
"thyroid pill." The thyroid gland furnishes thyroxin,
an important secretion for regulating body development and metabolism. But there's a "catch" in the use
of the thyroid pill—it stimulates the appetite as much
as it stimulates the metabolism, so that, although you
may burn up the food you eat faster, you're going to be
tempted to eat more.

According to Dr. Walter Modells, reporting on
the "Status and Prospect of Drugs for Overeating," the
thyroid pill, which has been in use for many years, will
result in a weight loss if the patient's diet can be
strictly limited, despite the stimulation of his appetite
by the drug. As he puts it, "Since obese patients have
difficulty in restraining their appetites under the best
of circumstances, most patients fail to limit their in-
take sufficiently |with the added stimulus to their ap-
petites provided by thyroid medication] to lose encouraging amounts of weight." Add to this the discomforts caused by the drug—"palpitations, warmth,
nervousness, insomnia, and excessive perspiration"—
plus the fact that the thyroid pill should not be used
for heart patients, and you have the sum of reasons
why it is unlikely that any individual will find the thyroid pill effective as a reducing agent for more than a
short time.

Just imagine the poor fat patient who, having put
his faith in thyroid drugs, wanders around the house
late at night, nervous and insomniac, hungrier than he

has ever been, trying to keep from raiding the refrigerator!

Perhaps a handy rule of thumb might be: any proposed weight control measure which *adds* to the great number of afflictions from which the obese already suffer ought to be seriously reconsidered . . . and, possibly, abandoned.

"But I Eat Like a Bird!"

Dr. Edgar S. Gordon, professor of medicine at the University of Wisconsin Medical School, indicates that there are at least 27 metabolic differences between obese and non-obese persons, although (thank heavens!) not all 27 differences are present in *every* case. Although it is the result of data gathered from several experimental laboratories, Dr. Gordon's conclusion that 25 percent of all obesity is due to metabolic disorders is not shared by everyone in the profession. There are still some authorities that don't believe that *any* case of obesity has a metabolic origin.

Since 1912, however, when William Osler, in his book *The Principles and Practice of Medicine,* defined obesity as a "disorder of metabolism," the general climate of opinion has been shifting toward the metabolic theory, at least as part of the picture. The unhappy victim of undue corpulence has, as a result, begun to receive sympathetic treatment rather than castigation for gluttony. It turns out that the portly matron who claims that she subsists on soda crackers and tea may be telling the truth, after all, and, however misguided her choice of diet, it has to be admitted that she hasn't been guilty of excessive eating.

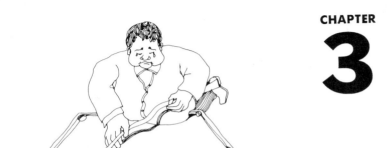

Has Heredity Put You behind the Eight Ball?

Just as it took a number of years for metabolic defects to be recognized as causes of obesity, many doctors have been reluctant to believe that a tendency toward obesity could be inherited. However, recent studies show that genetic factors may play a bigger role in certain cases of obesity than previously thought possible.

This means a tendency to store fat may be as much a part of an individual's inheritance as blue eyes or freckles. But, does this also mean that the person is a helpless victim of this legacy from his ancestors? Although the inheritors of a tendency to be obese must be vigilant about what they eat, no one who is selecting his own meals three times a day is helpless and hopeless. He may have to be more artful in that selection, more conscious of the nutritional value of different foods.

The tendency toward obesity is often compared to the tendency toward diabetes. According to Dr. Gordon, writing in *Postgraduate Medicine,* June, 1969, obesity and diabetes are practically first cousins anyway. Three metabolic errors seen in both diabetes and obesity support this concept: defective glucose metabolism, hyperinsulinism, and retention of water.

The normal person, says Dr. Gordon, burns the carbohydrate he eats—uses it up for energy. But not the obese person. He doesn't use carbohydrate for energy. He converts most of it into fat and stores the fat in rings and folds all over his body.

The forced accumulation of fat leads to the second metabolic defect—hyperinsulinism. The obese person shoots out up to ten times as much insulin as a normal person does after eating simple carbohydrate. The insulin rushes the sugar out of the bloodstream and into the cell, where it is stored as fat regardless of the body's actual need for fuel.

Water retention, a third diabetes-related defect, especially affects women. For every 100 grams of fat she loses, the obese woman retains 124 grams of water, at least in the beginning of her dieting regimen. It doesn't take a mathematician to observe that, at first, she will actually weigh more than she did before she gave up fattening foods. She is going to be a mighty discouraged gal unless she knows that this is a temporary setback. After three to six weeks, her system will become waterlogged and begin to release the excess fluid. (So, just hang in there, Baby!)

This phenomenon gave rise to one of the most

popular reducing drugs—diuretics, commonly called water pills. In helping to relieve the water-retention problem—which they do—diuretics also drain the system of potassium with a possible danger to the heart. Many expensive obesity "cures," that feature an amazing initial weight loss without dreary dieting, depend on diuretics to produce the "miracle" (otherwise known as dehydration).

The single important fact to remember is that loss of water is not a loss of fat—and excess fat is almost a definition of obesity. As soon as the client ceases to take the drugs, the water from the food she eats will begin to accumulate in her body and slimming Cinderella will have turned back into a chubby scullery maid!

A Few Facts and Figures about Figures and Fat

What's the likelihood of inherited obesity? A child with one obese parent is six times as likely to be obese as is a child with two non-obese parents. The likelihood becomes twelve to thirteen times greater if both of the child's parents are obese.

In experiments with mice, researchers found that mice prone to inherited obesity, had a metabolic defect that caused them to store much more fat than mice in a control group. The obese mice stored fat even while fasting! The elimination of certain food substances brought the weight down, but the mice held on to their fat so dearly that they remained obese in ratio to their total body composition. This is most likely true of people as well. Some experts say that about 10 percent of obesity cases appear to be related to inherited metabolic factors.

For some heavyweights, then, fat does "run in the family." While environmental conditions no doubt contribute to weight-gaining in some family situations— like being born into a family where *every* day is Prince Spaghetti Day—evidence indicates environmental influences alone do not explain the plight of those who lose weight only with great restraint and effort.

Dr. F. H. Wright, pediatrics expert at the University of Chicago, points out that, in a nursery for premature infants, where supervision and control are strict, where the environment is uniform for all infants, and detailed food-intake records are kept, "there is not an exact correlation for all infants between the amount of food consumed and the fatness which results." Even after other factors (the baby's display of activity and energy, the rate of growth, etc.) are accounted for, individual variations in how much and at what rate fat is stored remain. They can only be attributed to differences in the babies' physical constitutions.

Harvard's Dr. Jean Mayer reported, in *Clinical Nutrition*, April 1965, that research supports the theory that obesity runs in families. In studies of twins, the evidence on the importance of the genetic role in certain obesity cases seems even more definitive. If identical twins were reared and living in identical environments, the variation between them in body weight averaged a 1.39 percent difference. In dissimilar environments, the variation averaged 3.6 percent, which is still a very small amount. Although environment affects body weight to some degree, genetic factors are, according to Dr. Mayer, of "paramount importance."

One study showed that, in the pairing of parents who were both obese, three-fourths of the offspring were obese in the clinical sense. Matings of one obese and one non-obese parent produced obesity in 41 percent of the offspring. Non-obese parents brought forth only 9 percent obese offspring (and even that might be due to a fat forefather somewhere on the family tree).

Statistics vary, of course, from one study to another, but the indications are clear enough. If you don't want to be obese, you should have chosen skinny parents!

All right, then—since that's impossible, you *can* learn to recognize and understand your situation and to control the predispositions of your ancestry by wise nutritional eating habits. "Habit" can be a nasty word, if you think of it as something unpleasant imposed upon you from the outside. But if you think of it, instead, as your own decision, your own will, your own "whim" brought to the status of regular practice, it's really not such a bad word, after all! There can be a great deal of pleasure in the sense that you are controlling your own destiny, within the boundaries that nature has decreed.

Twiggy, Sophia, and Liz

Speaking of nature's boundaries—since there are people who may be structurally predisposed, even in favorable environmental situations, to be fatter than others, any systematic approach to the obesity problem must include a study of the morphological constitutions of obese persons. "Morphological" means form and structure as a whole—in other words, the way you "shape up."

In case you're a Scrabble or crossword buff, "somatotype" is the other important word here, and it means body type classification. Experts have defined body types in three categories: ectomorph, mesomorph, and endomorph. Although practically no one is a "pure" type, many people are predominantly one type or another. As you meet the three "morphys" in the following descriptions, perhaps you can spot the kind of body type that seems to fit you best.

If you're an ectomorph, your body is characterized by the predominance of the structures developed from the ectodermal (outer) layer of the embryo—skin, nerves, brain, and sense organs. You are probably lanky, thin, delicate in bone structure, and stringy in muscular development. You have long, slender fingers and toes. You're recognizable on the basis of linearity and fragility, meaning that you'll look svelte in just about anything you drape on your model's figure. Most important, it is doubtful that your reason for reading this book is to learn how to diet more effectively yourself, but rather to help someone you love attain that goal. Twiggy is predominantly an ectomorph.

If you're the athletic or muscular type, if your chest is massive and muscular and dominates over your abdomen, with strong muscular relief and prominent body joints, you're a mesomorph. Your body type is characterized by structures developed from the mesodermal (middle) layer of the embryo—muscle, bone, and connective tissue. You have broad shoulders, and your body tapers downward. Chances are you could become a first class swimmer, if you put your mind and muscle to it. People think twice before insulting or assaulting you. Some of you will have trouble controlling your weight, and some of you (not an overwhelming percentage) will be obese. If you're getting all the exercise you could with that excellent natural body equipment of yours, you can remain flat-bellied and trim on an ample diet. Sophia Loren is a mostly mesomorphic type.

Because the endomorph is the abdominal physical type, characterized by the structures developed from the endodermal (inner) layer of the embryo, this type of frame is predisposed to obesity. Here again, inheritance plays a part, because you inherit your somatotype tendencies from your parents. Many times this results in a nice mixture, but, if both your parents are endomorphs, you could be almost a "pure" type. In the endomorph, the abdomen mass overshadows the thoracic bulk (more belly than chest). The body's areas are notably soft and round. Hands and feet are relatively small with rather short fingers and toes. Your facial features, too, may be small and delicate. You are more often found sunning yourself on the deck of a boat than water skiing behind one. You prefer the museum or gourmet tour to the back-packing hike across Europe. You are, however, very, very huggable! Elizabeth Taylor is predominantly an endomorph.

What can one do about a body type? Some things a person just has to learn to live with! Endomorphs and mesomorphs will not be magically changed into ectomorphs no matter how many fashion magazines they study, admiring the angles and contortions of the lanky ectomorph models.

In choosing three lovely people as examples, perhaps the point is made that there's no need to yearn for a different somatotype than the one you have— and, indeed, it won't do you any good! But there is every reason to aspire to be a healthy, good-looking person of your own body type. A popular song states that "Everyone is beautiful in his own way . . ." Let's amend that to read, everyone *can be* beautiful in his own way.

Taking in more food of the wrong kinds than the body can use up in its daily activities is still the principle cause of overweight, but, if a person's body structure tends toward obesity, the need for caution and alertness is more critical. A healthful regimen seems less restrictive if a person understands as much as possible about the requirements of his own unique body.

As you can see, many factors, frequently in combination with each other, are responsible for obesity. Other factors work to camouflage or repress the tendency toward obesity: environmental conditions, and social and cultural pressures may support voluntary control of obesity, while scarce food supply and the need for heavy physical work may repress obesity tendencies automatically. Fashion is a great motivational factor. It is why so many persons in our time long for the super-slender, much-photographed ectomorphic body. But for a mesomorphic person to try dieting his way into this ideal is just as foolish as for him to permit his weight to become excessive through careless eating habits.

Not too fat nor too thin—but *just right* should be the goal of any diet or health regimen. Make that the standard by which you measure all fad diets which come to overnight fame in the pages of women's magazines. If the goals of a diet are fashion-dictated, if its aim is a quick, temporary reduction to show off your cheekbones (that wonderful gaunt look!)—it really is a waste of time and a risk of good health to pursue it.

Fat Cells Are Stranger Than Fiction

Several authorities say that children with an obesity potential will increase the number of their fat cells during their early weight-gaining phases. Although later dieting may cause a loss of the fat itself, it will not decrease the number of storage cells for fat. In other words, the fat cells will shrink, but they'll still *be* there.

Conversely, there are cases in which middle-aged people, who were slim in their early years, suddenly put on a great deal of weight. This was due to the increased size of their existing fat cells, but not their number. A good weight-reducing regimen will shrink the enlarged fat cells, and these individuals will have an easier time maintaining the loss than will those who, early in life, increased their fat storage potential with an excess number of fat cells.

These facts have given rise to two of the strangest concepts in the annals of obesity literature: thin obesity and fat non-obesity. Let us attempt to explain in the simplest terms possible, before total confusion reigns!

Suppose you were a chubby child of whom everyone said, "what a cutie-pie—I just love pinching those fat little legs!" If you hollered while being stuffed with goodies by your mother you had every right to object, because you weren't getting healthier—you were just increasing the number of fat storage cells in your roly-poly little body. Okay—so, later on, you got away from Mom's apple pie and dieted yourself into a lovely trim shape. You got rid of the fat bulges, yet you're a "thin obese" person, and you're going to have to guard that great new figure especially well to maintain it.

Suppose, on the other hand, you were a skinny little kid, much to your mother's chagrin. She may even have called you a "feeding problem," and there was much hushed consultation between your mother and her friends over the matter. After a number of years, some change in your life style brought on a substantial weight gain. Perhaps you married a French pastry chef, or broke your leg while skiing in the Alps, or both. Whatever the reason—too much food or too little exercise—you found yourself several sizes bigger than you desired. True, you increased the amount of fat in your body, but not the amount of fat storage cells. That was set at a low number back when you were a youngster. So now you can be considered a fat non-obese person, because, once you lose the excess poundage, you're not going to have to contend with a large number of fat cells.

As long as you're slim, what do you care if you're a case of thin obesity or thin non-obesity? What's in a name anyway?

Maintenance of your correct weight is why you care. The clinically obese, whether currently fat or thin as of this reading, have a greater capacity to synthesize and store fat and a greater need for dietary caution.

Riding on a Vicious Cycle

Reporting on the results of recent observations of these matters, Dr. Gordon says, not only are there more fat cells in clinically obese persons, but the fat cells are larger and greedier for glucose. Glucose circulating in the bloodstream is quickly absorbed into these cells and converted into fat, despite the fact that this may leave your blood short of glucose. To supply needed energy, the fat cells flood the bloodstream with fatty acids. This excess of fatty acids in the blood, in turn, makes it still more difficult for your system to burn glucose, which is again stored as fat instead. A vicious cycle is established and maintained, to the eternal frustration of the clinically obese.

At this point the kind of food eaten becomes more important than the amount. Carbohydrates are the villains here, and, if you're clinically obese, a diet whose only restriction is in the number of calories you consume daily will have to be dangerously low to work for you. That neat little calorie guide booklet you bought at the checkout counter of your supermarket, which lists 37 kinds of candy and 24 varieties of cookies, is not exactly putting you on, but it's not presenting you with the complete picture either. Nowhere in that book does it say that sugar and starches are your enemies.

Improving Your Mathematical Skills

Heredity plays a role in determining how a person's body uses the food he eats; there are several measurable differences between the obese and the non-obese. One person's rate of calorie absorption may be different from another's, for example, which is why counting calories may improve your arithmetic, but is hardly an efficient measurement of your body's actual use of food. The rate at which those calories become hormones, enzymes, or blood cells, are oxidized as free fatty acids, stored as fat, burned up in activity, or disposed as waste, *varies* from one person to another.

Not only does absorption of calories differ from one person to another, but it varies in the same person from time to time. It is these differences in calorie utilization that cast doubt upon any standard calorie tables for general application.

So, if your ancestors have passed on to you, along with curly hair and a talent for playing the piano, the propensity for obesity, you have every reason in the world to take extra precaution with your food habits. You need to understand what your body is liable to do, check on that natural tendency toward fat storage, and eat sensibly so that your body receives the nourishment it requires without adding to its "fat bank." Increase your opportunities for exercise and activity, and enjoy life as if you had no more problems than the svelte blonde in the next apartment (who can't play a note and whose hair is limp, anyway!)

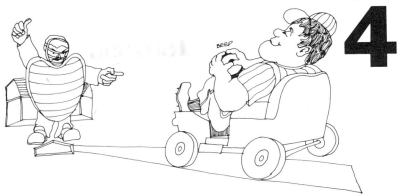

You're Out!—You're Not Playing the Game

Civilization and industrialization have done wonderful things for you. Now you can go up the down staircase by escalator, drive your 427 horsepower to the corner store for milk, compact your trash into one easy trip, and beat your cake batter with an electric whisk. With all these "wonders," it's a wonder that you have to get out of bed at all! Unfortunately, this "saving" of your precious energy may be deposited directly into your "fat bank."

You don't gain weight just by overeating. Even if you've been lithe and lissome in the past, as you get older, your level of physical activity tends to diminish. Unless you limit the contents of your meals accordingly, you run the risk of becoming overweight.

"But I eat just like I always have." Yes, and do

you move around as much as you always have?—or are you becoming a "fat cat" with an electrical appliance for every chore, even brushing your teeth and combing your hair?

In addition to the lure of the "easy life," the older person tends to adopt sedentary habits (otherwise known as "getting into a rut") that preclude the sports and games he used to enjoy—a long swim, a fast polka, a hike through bird-watching country, a romp with someone of the opposite sex. Too frequently the middle-aged person depends upon TV to supply life's excitement. From dinnertime until sleepy-time, he is liable to sit and sip and nibble and watch, a vicarious adventurer.

The obese person is often like one prematurely aged, in that he has even less inclination for exercise than the non-obese individual. Pedometer tests have shown that obese women walk an average of under two miles a day compared to four and one-half miles for their normal-weight sisters. Obese men walk about three and one-quarter miles, while men of normal weight average six and one-fifth miles a day.

Studies reveal that, although the obese child's food consumption is usually equal to or below the food consumption of normal children, the chubby youngsters are much less active, exercising only about one-third as much as their thinner friends. And even that activity is performed with as little effort as they can manage.

Researchers at the University of Wisconsin have found that people whose weight is 50 percent fat have less than half the maximum work capacity of people with 12 percent fat. In normal-sized men, oxygen pressures between capillaries and lung air sacs are equal.

In obese men, these pressures are decidedly different, indicating that oxygen isn't getting across the lung membrane very easily. Therefore, the extra oxygen necessary for exercising is obtained with greater difficulty. Excess fat layers seem to weigh upon the diaphragm, making it harder to inflate the lungs. The energy required for any kind of motion increases as the available oxygen decreases.

Much as we deplore the prejudice against hiring the obese (a prejudice that groups like the NAAFA— the National Association to Aid Fat Americans, Inc.— may be applauded for fighting) this diminished work capacity does not encourage employers to fill open positions on their staff with the slow-moving, fat applicant.

The joyless prospect for the very overweight person is that, while his size makes exercise burdensome, insufficient exercise encourages deposits of additional fat. The onset of overweight can often be traced to a decrease in physical activity—and another vicious cycle begins to roll!

Even if one cuts down food intake to a calorie level which should make it impossible to gain weight, at least some physical activity is essential to maintain a healthy, well-toned body. It's amazing but true that even a size-eight female can develop flab around her middle in the middle years, which prevents her from wearing certain tucked-in blouses that she would like to wear, and a certain looseness around the underarm that suddenly convinces her that longer sleeves are more becoming.

The best exercise is the one you enjoy and are capable of doing well. The best way to build up your muscle tone is *slowly*.

A physical culture expert who puts you through a series of arduous calisthenics that bore you and leave you aching in every limb is not doing you a favor. You're better off to make a game of exercise or go dancing for your exercise, if dancing is something you really like to do. For one thing, you're liable to continue to seek a pleasant experience. For another, life is to be enjoyed, not postponed until a later date. The happier you are, the easier it will be to organize your eating habits in a more healthful way.

If, on the other hand, you loathe dancing and find calisthenics relaxing after a hard day at the office, by all means take up a moderate program of "bends" and "lifts." The message here is do *something,* do it *sensibly,* and enjoy yourself while you're at it.

How easily the decrease in activity sneaks into one's life! Strange, because a lot of good fun is replaced by stagnation in the process. Collecting shells on the beach is infinitely more exciting than buying them in a gift shop.

A nice balance between increased activity and healthful, slimming meals can slowly and pleasantly put you on the road to normal weight. One remedy cannot function adequately without the other.

Notable among the misleading applications of exercise is Dr. Abraham L. Friedman's book *How Sex Can Keep You Slim.* Truly, if you want to sell a book, you can't do better than to combine the subjects of overweight and sex. But the principle behind Dr. Friedman's message—reach for your mate instead of your plate—is emphasizing one important, but *only* one, aspect of life to the exclusion of others. Sex is a calorie-consuming activity. It is enjoyable but, within the limits of reason, it is not *enough* activity to keep you thin. A new mealtime regimen and an increase in other (perhaps more mundane) activites as well will also be required. As a substitute for food, sexual activity will only work for a limited time. Even honeymooners eventually go out of the hotel for hamburgers and more champagne. Dr. Friedman has a fun idea there, but it's a little naive and, at times, could be somewhat inconvenient to practice.

Obesity and Its Evil Companions

While the person of normal weight can, at age 45, look forward to about 25 more years of fruitful living, the person who is 30 percent overweight can expect to close his account at the "fat bank" in about 12 years. Excess weight is a killer. This is a sobering statistic, but it has to be faced. And no organ or part of the body is hurt more by obesity than the heart. Associated diseases and disorders spring up like weeds in an untended garden.

In Germany, the incidence of high blood pressure is up 250 percent since World War II. High blood pressure, along with other coronary illnesses, accounts for 40 percent of all German deaths, according to Dr. Rausch, head of the Federal Republic's Food Council. Obesity is a major factor and, "The wrong diet is as much involved in the prevalence of heart disorders as the stresses of business life," says Dr. Rausch.

"We have a new epidemic," said Dr. Vaeinoe Soininen, medical officer of Finland's North Karelia County where the unusually high incidence of heart attacks has led to a five-year experiment which involves

186,000 Finns. Researchers are working on the theory that the cause is the environment—chiefly the diet and smoking. The North Karelian diet is high in dairy fats and contains few vegetables.

The overweight population of America dies from heart disease at three times the rate of the underweight population, and twice the rate of those of normal weight.

Although blood pressure rises as weight rises, this damaging effect of obesity *is reversible* when the weight is trimmed. Reducing weight reduces blood pressure and spares the heart correspondingly. This is certainly one of the most "heartening" facts about obesity. The day you begin to direct your body toward normal weight is the day you will also begin your recuperation from the attendant health problems of obesity.

One such problem is hypometabolism (a low rate of metabolic activity), a constant companion to obesity. This abnormality has a direct effect on many body components and on the manner in which they function, develop, and maintain themselves. In a recent East German study of 1,000 obese subjects, 752 women and 248 men, almost 20 percent, showed signs of hypertension. Over half the subjects suffered from coronary insufficiency, which occurs when the heart is not able to pump sufficient blood through the body for optimum health. A correlation between the presence of hypertension and the age and *degree* of obesity in the subject was shown. There was also a definite relationship between the presence of coronary insufficiency and the subjects' ages and weights. In other words, a little fat is healthier than a lot of fat. Which means it's better for you to reduce *some* of your weight than not to reduce at all.

Hyperinsulinism, water retention (mostly in women) and diabetes are other disorders which commonly accompany obesity, as already noted.

The overweight person, then, has a double purpose in establishing for himself an intelligent program of weight reduction—not only to extend life, but also to live those years as vigorously as possible, free of the many "ills" that afflict the obese.

If the "settling years" tend to make you want to slow down, let a degree of awareness of these very real and evil companions of overweight motivate you toward keeping trim and active. You'll enjoy life more and like yourself better without that "middle-aged spread."

We offer this little folk-verse to recite to yourself, especially on birthdays:

> EAT LESS; BREATHE MORE.
> TALK LESS; THINK MORE.
> RIDE LESS; WALK MORE.
> CLOTHE LESS; BATHE MORE.
> WORRY LESS; WORK MORE.
> WASTE LESS; GIVE MORE.
> PREACH LESS; PRACTICE MORE.

The View from the Family Album

Dr. Williams, in his book, *Nutrition Against Disease,* supports the theory that some obese persons are victims of hereditary factors. Dr. George Edward Schauff, in a paper explaining the QQF theory (Quality and Quantity of Food Plus Frequency of Ingestion) claims that "the seeds of the predisposition toward obesity are planted very early in life."

If only you could travel backwards in some marvellous time machine to change your own metabolic patterns! (The wonder is that some reducing salon has not yet offered such a machine to their gullible clients.) But, since you have to work with the natural laws as they govern your own individual development to the age you are now, it can only be suggested that parents recognize the potential problem of obesity in their children and thus help to spare them the later frustrations of an obese metabolism. We can see that there are warning signs: in family history, in bodily structure and in early chubbiness, so mistakenly seen as "cute." If there seems to be a definite danger, extra care can be taken that the child's everyday meals do not include foods which contribute to obesity rather than to good nutrition.

Since many of our "tastes" in food are also established in those first years, the subtle influence of a home where fresh ripe peaches are served for dessert rather than peach pie and whole wheat toast is offered for a snack instead of chocolate cookies can remain as a benefit for life. Such influences improve metabolic patterns and initiate a "taste" for the healthier foods that will not require any sharp reversals later on.

Alexander Bell, the Wright Brothers, et al

Man has displayed his amazing adaptive ingenuity in many fields. He can hear what's being said hundreds of miles away, fly though he hasn't wings, probe the depths of the sea although he is basically a land animal, see through microscopes and telescopes what can't be seen by the naked eye, and correct all manner of physical deficiencies with clever gadgets such as eyeglasses and hearing aids. He is learning to influence such hitherto implacable forces as the weather and natural selection—and, someday, no doubt, will be able to "leap tall buildings with a single bound."

But he can't seem to master this basic matter of weight control. Hopefully, the realization that an obese person may be as much a victim of his condition as he is its agent will increase chances for more serious and successful efforts at control. How far better and easier to correct overweight before it becomes a matter of controlling diabetes, high blood pressure, or heart disease.

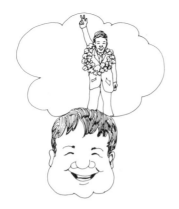

Think Thin and Win

Hunger is the very first tension-producing experience in our lives. Within a few hours after being born, the infant wants food—and becomes tense until his hunger is satisfied. This tension is both life-giving and disturbing. Some researchers theorize that it could help to account for the basic fear of starvation which we may carry with us into adulthood.

Speculation does not stop with these observable phenomena, however, but also delves into the early ages of the species of man. Dr. Theodore B. Van Italie of Columbia University says the tendency to overeat is normal. Until recent times, according to this line of thought, man's food supply came when he was lucky enough to catch and kill it—which happened a lot less often than you are able to raid the meat counter at the supermarket. To survive between successful hunts, our ancestors gorged themselves whenever possible, not just to satisfy hunger, but to store up against the day of famine. Thus man is conditioned to overeat.

Yet Doctors James H. Hutton and Angelo P. Creticos, in an article published in *Industrial Medicine And Surgery,* point out that obesity was "non-existent prior to the inauguration of regular meals . . . In pre-neolithic times, man ate only when he was hungry and only as much as was needed to satisfy his hunger." The article goes on to support the theory that continual nibbling was our original meal plan and the one to which our digestive tract is best adjusted.

If, at this juncture, you're beginning to feel some vague confusion, this is a good place to point out one of the more challenging aspects of our current obesity shelf in the library—*"experts" do not agree!* "You pays your money and you takes your choice," as the saying goes, and nowhere is that truer than in a review of psychological factors in obesity.

Whatever the dining peccadillos of Mr. Preneolithic Man, it appears that we can't depend on the caveman's life style to explain away current obesity problems, any more than he can be used for an excuse for us to drag our mate off to a cave by the hair. Therefore, we offer these psychological studies and speculations in the interest of presenting all aspects of the problem of obesity and not to foster the ever-easy "just can't help myself" philosophy.

Many psychological factors which are thought to influence obesity have only recently been researched, and the very contemporaneity of these studies suggests that there is much territory still to be explored. Yet, from these uncharted areas, we can glimpse new directions and awareness that can be of help to an overweight person, if they are used to encourage, rather than to discourage, progress toward better health.

"I'm in the Mood for Food"

It's become generally apparent that emotions play an important part in obesity. Many overweight people eat more when they are under stress, although the opposite is true of underweight individuals. Stress, therefore, seems to exaggerate whatever food-related tendencies are already present.

Human beings are not built of separate compartments. Body processes affect moods and emotions; mental and emotional processes affect the body. When you harbor anxiety, fear, or hostility, there is little question but that these emotions, probably by hormonal mechanisms, alter the microenvironment of the cells which make up the appestat.

Certain life experiences are continually cited as stepping stones to obesity: a change of job, especially from one requiring considerable physical exertion to a "step up the ladder" desk job; a change of environment, particularly if you move from where food is plain and scarce to where it is plentiful and sophisticated; having an acute or serious infection that may influence the hypothalamus; an emotional trauma such as the dissolution of a love affair or the death of a loved one.

It has also been suggested that individuals overeat and become obese because they are bored, unloved, insecure, or under tension. There is, regrettably, no practical means for avoiding such feelings.

Many obese persons whose lives will be shortened by their condition nevertheless are reluctant or refuse to alter their life style with regard to food intake and exercise. They can appreciate the seriousness of oncoming diabetes, hypertension, heart disease—all the usual complications of obesity—and they are often of high intelligence, but even a combination of diet and psychotherapy may not produce the necessary changes in eating habits.

It has been the clinical experience of Doctors Hutton and Creticos that patients who are particularly fond of the carbohydrate foods will have the most difficult time dieting successfully. This is an interesting point and, if you are a dieter who relishes cakes, pies, pizza, and spaghetti, what hope is held out to you? Should you just quit dieting and accept your fat fate?

There is hope, but you won't find it in most medical literature about obesity, which continually admits failure to produce permanent weight losses. Instead, you're going to have to look within yourself for qualities (admittedly abstract) like confidence in your ability to change and faith in your future goals. Even something as highly personal as tastes in food can be changed.

Here's one line of reasoning you can follow: a predilection for certain rare foods is known as an "acquired taste"—you know, like black olives or smoked fish or Camembert cheese. A two-year-old is likely to spit them out instantly as unfit for human consumption. Somewhere along the line, people learn to enjoy the flavor and texture of these and other "gourmet" foods, but it takes effort and persistence. After you get the first raw oyster down, for instance, you have to be willing to try another . . . and another. If you've finally become an oyster-on-the-half-shell devotee, you can take a certain pride in it. (After all, some folks never make it!) Consider that the same process is at work in substituting a taste for lean broiled meat and fresh melon in place of lasagna and apple fritters. You have to expect it to take time and patience.

If you're dieting, hunger will be on your side, so that dinner is liable to look and smell delicious even if it isn't fortified by mashed potatoes and pecan rolls. You can gradually *de-acquire* your taste for foods which are personally anathema to your body—but you have to *believe* that you can!

Gluttony is the only one of the Seven Deadly Sins which harms no one but yourself, says N. W. Pirie in an article in the *New Scientist,* calling it "a personal matter." The unseen consequences of sin (if this be sin) are subtle, though. What about the harm gluttony does to the family who loves—and may lose—the rampant trencherman?

Some experts, frustrated by the failure of information campaigns on the dangers of obesity to motivate individuals toward more rapid and consistent weight loss, have voiced the doubt that people really want to prolong their life span appreciably. Dr. Rulson of Harvard has commented wryly, "if we rule out obesity as a cause of death, we'll be forty years on pensions." Not exactly an upbeat view of the "age of serenity!"

Obviously, ways must be found to mobilize self-interest and the desire to enjoy the pleasures of every stage of life in order to effectively combat the obesity problem.

To say that every extremely obese person has a psychological need to remain in an overweight condition is a debatable and not very helpful generalization. Nevertheless, some doctors consider obesity almost completely a psychological problem and feel that attempts to reduce will not succeed until underlying emotional difficulties are solved. In answer, we suggest that life can be so much more pleasant, emotionally as well as physically, for the person who achieves normal weight, and this, in itself, can relieve some of his psychological problems.

Food, the psychologists say, is used by some as a substitute for family or sexual affection; for others, obesity is a shield used to ward off advances by the opposite sex. Food can provide a shell into which a person retreats to avoid competition and possible failure or mature responsibility. Obesity may be a self-punishment or a repression of hostility against a parent or spouse.

In *Diet Is Not Enough,* Dr. Irving B. Perlstein and William Cole declare that "because of improper training early in life or the inability to cope with some difficulty in their personal relationships or environment, they (the overeaters) use food for emotional purposes. Thousands use narcotics to anesthetize their anxieties and conflicts. Millions use alcohol. Tens of millions resort to food—a sedative that is cheaper, more available, and far more respectable."

Other physicians, however, point out that emotional problems may *result* from obesity rather than be its cause. The question as posed to *you* is: did anxiety drive you into consuming too many hot fudge sundaes or did the bulging results of too many sundaes make you unduly anxious and tense? Before you really get hung up on that one, here's another: what are you going to *do* about it?

"I Ate It Because It Was There"

A revealing experiment in external stimulation on the obese used "feeding machines" filled with a nutritious but rather tasteless substance which could be eaten by the overweight and normal subjects at any time of the day or night they wished. The normal weight subjects (whatever their private feelings about the chef) ate sufficient calories each day to maintain their weight. Surprisingly, obese subjects ate very little, so little, in fact, that they lost weight, although they were encouraged to "help themselves." Taking the joy out of eating succeeded where many other methods failed.

Obese persons, it seems, have lost their internal caloric sense, and, if the food is unattractive and unappetizing, they eat less than they need to maintain weight. If, on the other hand, the cook lays out a complete holiday dinner with all the trimmings, every course perfectly cooked and beautifully presented, the obese person is the one who isn't going to know when to quit, and, even when the food has been put away, will be out in the kitchen looking for a turkey sandwich. Such people lack a good braking system to tell them when to stop eating, providing the food itself is pleasing.

Dr. Stanley Schechter, a social psychologist at Columbia University, said ". . . the overweight person literally may not know when he is physiologically hungry." Apparently, people who are overweight do not recognize "hunger" by the same set of bodily symbols as normal-weight persons do. Hunger is to them what they feel when they see a tray of French pastries passing by. That's different from the signal bodies give when food is needed for energy to perform tasks.

Of course, everyone is influenced to some extent by external cues in eating. The good smells of herbs and onions, the taste of a favorite roast, the sight of other people enjoying dinner—these are all cues that function independently of the pure hunger state. But, for the obese, all cues seem to be working. The internal "turn off" to food is barely perceived. The normal-weight person may be influenced by external cues, but he is also very much aware of the internal signals about the actual state of his stomach.

Other tests have shown that manipulating clocks so that they move faster through the hours will bring the obese person to the table that much sooner, whereas the normal-weight person waits until his stomach (not the clock on the wall) says "lunch time."

In other studies, large trays of before-dinner snacks were offered to subjects for nibbling. The normal-weight persons did not wish "to spoil dinner," but obese subjects evidently did not think they were in that danger. They knew they could eat lots of yummy canapes and *hors d'oeuvres,* and a large dinner, as well.

Shall the obese person remove himself from all temptation, then—forbid the odor of baking bread, turn off the television during ice cream commercials, refuse to pass restaurants and hamburger stands, choosing devious routes through town to avoid them, so that he will be less inclined to crave food? This would work, for a time, but once the sensory-limitation regimen was over, he would be right back in The Garden of Eden again, reaching for an apple pie.

It appears that the conscious, logical decision of the obese person's intellect must do what the involuntary signals from the body won't do. He must make up his mind not to seek out known temptations, and not to flee from life either.

Having the refrigerator stocked with the right kinds of foods instead of the fattening ones can be a start. One neat rationalization to *avoid* this elementary solution is "consideration" for the other members of one's family. But, when you get right down to it, raw fruits and vegetables and lean meats won't hurt the other members of the family one bit. Chances are people of normal weight won't even notice the missing cookie jar. Nutritious substitutes can be provided, and everyone's health will be improved while the obese person has less temptation to stray from the path of his diet. After all, families share, by their very union, many other states in common—their income, their neighborhood, an extra-large backyard, or a lack of closet space. So, too, they can share in helping their obese member to attain a healthier weight.

Everyone in the family should have the same menu at dinner, even if only one person is dieting. It is unreasonable to expect a dieter to be satisfied with four ounces of cottage cheese when everyone else is having chicken pot pie. Better that the whole family share a meal of broiled chicken and steamed vegetables. (The use of the right herbs can make this into a gourmet treat.)

Once upon a time, the housewife could only buy

as much food as she could carry home and store. Now we have supermarkets, and stationwagons, plus additional freezer space and shelf space galore. Even if a woman takes her husband with her, they will probably come out of the market with more food than they can carry by themselves. Furthermore, it's considered by many an intolerable chore, but a necessity, to stock up thus for the week.

Perhaps a giant step backwards is in order. Most families have too many high-caloried snacks around the house anyway, which are parcelled out to the children in place of time and affection. "Don't cry. Mommy will give you a cup cake." And Mother will probably have one herself, "just for energy." If you or some member of your family is obese, it's time to give serious reconsideration to buying habits and menu-planning. Chances are, *everyone* will profit from it.

"Mirror, Mirror on the Wall..."

Psychological difficulties for the obese do not necessarily end with successful reducing. Even after losing a good many pounds, some dieters are unable to "see" themselves as thinner, according to some surprising experiments conducted by Dr. Jules Hirsh at Rockefeller University. Using a device that enabled him to project fatter and thinner "versions" of his patients' silhouettes onto a screen, Dr. Hirsh asked each subject to select the figure that most closely corresponded to his own. His patients still "saw" themselves in their former chubby proportions.

"It may be simply that they've been fat for so long that it takes a long time to readjust their thinking," suggests Dr. Hirsh, "but we prefer to think it is something special, perhaps biochemical." He hopes his experiment will help to explain why fat people almost always regain the weight they lose. (The insanities of many diet regimens may help to explain that one. Small wonder that the dieter can hardly wait to get off something like the lettuce and tomato semi-starvation diet, total 445 calories a day, and back to "normal" meals.)

Dr. Hirsh claims that the "body-image studies," which were accomplished with the help of Dr. Joel Grinker and Dr. Myron Glucksman, indicate that the central nervous system has a memory of its own.

Tests which involve the sense of time have also been made. A group of fat and thin subjects were asked to guess whether a series of recorded sounds lasted more or less than one second. All subjects averaged about the same number of correct answers. However, when the obese subjects had reduced, they erred on the high side, imagining that the sounds lasted longer than they really did. Dr. Hirsh believes these experiments may help to explain why formerly fat patients move slowly and exhibit a general apathy.

In general, fat people regard their proportions with disfavor, while the victims of anorexia (the inability to eat a sufficient amount of food, through a pathological failure of appetite) often find the condition of emaciation beautiful.

Self-image, to be sure, is a problem area to the obese—and so is the image they project to others, especially in this era when the painfully-thin female is exhibited in magazines as a desirable example to all. Some spunky heavy-weights have banded together to combat what they believe to be rank prejudice against them, voicing a resentment of job discrimination and other, more subtle, forms of intollerance. They speak out against the vogue for leanness, the government's physical fitness programs, and the amount of time which the media devote to the ideal of thinness—all those diet drink commercials, for instance. They counter with a "fat is beautiful" campaign which appears to serve to keep up the spirits of their rotund ranks.

The National Association to Aid Fat Americans (NAAFA) describes itself as an organization to "increase the happiness and well-being of overweight Americans," which is certainly a laudable aim. But, unfortunately, it is also increasing the general atmosphere of hopelessness that pervades the fat condition already, and they are de-emphasizing the health danger involved in obesity.

This attitude may make everyone feel better for a short time. But the fat person knows he has difficulty moving around and just catching his breath, no matter what slogans he repeats to himself.

Lew Louderback is another well-known advocate of the fat-is-fine image. "More people *should* be fat" is his contention, and he points out all the failures of medicine to "cure" obesity, along with the dangers of dieting itself, physical and emotional.

For example, Dr. Clifford F. Castineau of the Mayo Clinic is quoted: "It is probable that many extremely obese persons subconsciously make the choice to remain fat because of the emotional advantage offered by their adiposity. Overeating may be a means of releasing simple nervous tension in some persons, but in other persons, overeating and obesity may be an important defense against destructive emotional forces."

Dieting may unleash these forces. Dr. Albert J. Stunkard of the University of Pennsylvania states that more than one out of three patients in a control group suffered "severe emotional upsets" while dieting.

Although some depressed people have anorexia and weigh less, others eat *more* to lift themselves out of depressed states and to quiet anxiety, finding in food a special comfort. However, continuous weight gains will usually plunge them ever deeper into emotional problems as they are forced to deal with the realities of disfigurement and lack of mobility. Yet, these very drawbacks may provide excuses for avoiding social contacts that are actually the source of embarrassment and fear. As we have seen, there is more than one vicious cycle in the fields of fatness.

Many doctors suggest that obesity is incurable.

This is a side of the coin that should be viewed, especially if you are contemplating a "crash diet" to rid yourself of a weight build-up that has taken place over many years. We suggest that a whole, healthful change of life-style, involving a slow but lasting weight loss, makes a lot more sense than a miracle diet. We *don't* agree that abandoning hope of ever losing weight is the answer, nor is convincing yourself that your plight is really what you want anyway. If it's taken you an appreciable time to gain the extra pounds, you can allow for a longer amount of time to lose them. Even if you never go back to the weight you consider ideal, *any* weight loss will be to the benefit of your health and your enjoyment of life. Of course, nothing succeeds like success, and, once you've proved to yourself what you can do, you may be inspired to do more.

Some doctors insist upon a visit to a psychologist before beginning a diet regimen, and, frequently, patients will complain of many problems without mentioning their all too obvious fatness. Psychologists believe that the more a patient minimizes the reality of obesity, the more he is in need of psychological counselling.

We need a system like that of Alcoholics Anonymous. A very overweight person ought to be able to stand up and say "I am obese," realize the truth of it, and get ready to make some changes.

"Eat Fast, or You'll Fast"

Many overweight people get into the habit of eating at top speed. It may be a method of getting the most hot biscuits and pieces of fried chicken, in case there aren't any more in the kitchen. Or a sleight-of-hand whereby one appears to have eaten less because of taking less time to do it. Or just because, with his higher base line of adipose tissue (fat cells), the chubby person is the hungriest come meal time. Professor Richard E. Nesbett of the University of Michigan has been studying the similarities between fat people and hungry people, and he claims the obese "eat more because they are genuinely hungrier than persons of normal weight."

The speed at which food is eaten does make a difference to the dieter. In one experiment, rats in one cage were given their daily allowance of food during a two-hour period, while rats in another cage were allowed to nibble their ration over a 24-hour span. The forced fast-eaters soon became the fattest rats in the lab, even though the *amount* of food they were given was the same.

Not only will slowing down the pace of your meals help you to lose weight, but there are certain side benefits to be gained. If your dinner lasts an hour instead of ten minutes, you're more likely to feel a certain psychological satiety, because you've dined, with a capital D. It will be a lot better for your digestion than gobbling. Dinner table conversation flourishes when the pace is slower, and it looks a bit nicer to take small bites and chew them carefully. Fast eaters will really have to concentrate, though, to accomplish this one.

Secret eating binges are another habit to be resisted by the dieter who wants to be successful. Some rotund individuals don't eat very much when others are watching at meal times, but just give them five minutes alone in the kitchen! Cold cuts disappear like magic, pies shrink to a sliver, and it's obvious that the "milk and cookie monster" has been on the prowl again. These secret raids allow the fat folk to perpetuate certain useful myths: the notion that they don't eat much but, for some strange reason, their diet just doesn't work right, and the idea that those extra calories won't really turn into extra pounds. This last bit of self-fooling is a little irrational, and, sometimes, this kind of denial reaches psychotic proportions. That's why writing down every morsel you eat is such a good way of seeing your eating habits in an objective way. You won't have to do it forever—just long enough to see where you're going wrong.

"Night eating" is another habit to which the obese are often addicted. Sometimes this practice is the result of their attempts to diet, if the diet consists of cutting down on the number of meals per day. By some obscure process of reasoning, it always seems easier to begin by eliminating breakfast. Most people feel rushed in the morning or would rather sleep fifteen minutes more than eat. But breakfast is an important source of energy for the day. Still, overweight people often take pride in how little they eat in the morning. The "just coffee" person tops the "juice and coffee" breakfaster, while the chubby gal who skips lunch, too, is one up on them both. She is unmindful that these two meals provide important fuel for the day's work and play.

People on this sort of "diet" usually admit to what they modestly call "one good meal a day," which they enjoy just as they are ready to fall into a chair in front of TV. Often this meal is fortified by a bedtime snack that would have done justice to King Henry VIII. In these two feedings, more food is consumed than most people of normal weight eat in three meals during the day.

Taste buds are a little sluggish in the morning, but they're easily titillated at night. Also, food eaten just before bed has a maternal comfort that appeals to the lonely and anxious. Whatever the reason, "night eating" and concentrating food intake into a short span of time promotes the storage of fat.

Parents who lay down the law "clean your plate, or else" may be beginning a lifelong habit that will trigger obesity in those with the potential for it. With this kind of early training, the well-behaved fatty may continue to eat everything in sight like a "good boy," even when "everything" is a whole basket of white bread served with a mammoth bowl of spaghetti. And that's just the first course.

At some ages, it is necessary to take more precautions against weight gain than at others. Puberty is such an age in both sexes. A child may have been a finicky eater age three and the subject of much parental urging to "eat up," but if they're still pushing the potatoes and butter when the child has become a rotund thirteen, it's time to reappraise and update the advice.

Gluttony is a phenomenon that has few counterparts among wild animals. Barnyard animals, of course, may get as fat as their masters, either through enforced idleness or by the design of those who intend to profit by the pound at the marketplace. Steers are deliberately fattened while penned, food is stuffed into the throats of pinioned geese, and lights are snapped on in the middle of the night at the henhouse so that chickens will eat more—otherwise, these animals would be guided by instinct to maintain a proper weight. Hibernation, metamorphosis, will cause certain animals to consume extra calories, but all for a purpose, to provide for a necessary fast and a new stage of growth. Except for these physiological crises, animals follow the instincts with which nature has endowed them to seek a normal weight.

Overeating, "stuffing," gluttony—these can be a form of "showing off," of being the undisputed blueberry-pie-eating champion at the county fair or the best and biggest gourmet on the block, but, more often, it is a habit pattern begun when an individual was young with an exuberant metabolism and an active life. In later life, when he neither circulates as enthusiastically nor produces the same internal heat, when he is all bundled up by the fireplace in cold weather instead of out ice-skating in a lightweight turtleneck sweater, eating patterns that were once reasonable have now become excessive.

Hypnosis is a technique which has been used by psychologists and doctors to change unhealthy eating habits, but with limited success. First of all, hypnosis should never be attempted by any but qualified persons, since psychological disturbance can result. Secondly, not everyone can be hypnotized. It takes both concentration and trust in the hypnotist to accomplish this state.

A case was once reported in which a woman sent her husband to a doctor to be hypnotized. The husband had a habit of grinding his teeth in his sleep, which disturbed her rest. In a way, sessions were successful. As a result of post-hypnotic suggestions, the husband *did* stop grinding his teeth at night. But now he tried to strangle his wife in his sleep instead! Obviously, the problem was deeply rooted and had many unknown ramifications.

Self-help books on the subject of hypnotism, and especially self-hypnotism, outline programs whereby you can cure yourself of everything from obesity to impotency. Self-hypnotism is a method of getting in touch with your own unconscious mind. This is neither as weird as it sounds nor as effective as the book jacket would lead you to believe. Chances are the untrained layman will achieve only the lightest of hypnotic states —or just fall asleep!

The purpose of self-hypnosis in dieting is to program yourself to successful reducing and to discourage poor eating habits. The failure of the conscious mind to summon up sufficient "will power" will be corrected by the aid of the unconscious mind, something like sending to the fort for the cavalry. Such a move is for desperate predicaments only, as all movie fans know. If your diet is a sensible, nutritious, and reasonably filling one, you really won't be overwhelmed by impossible odds anyway.

Second only to sex, eating habits give the most private kind of enjoyment and are the most firmly fixed of personality traits in the opinion of many psychologists. These are emotional habits about which people prefer not to be lectured. They will not be forced to restrain them by an unctuous lot of evangelists who have never experienced the woes and pleasures of the transgressing overeater. That's why self-motivation and self-imposed corrective patterns are most likely to last for a lifetime. We hope to help overweight persons respond healthfully to their own unique situations, without resorting to the "sensational" regimens, whose effectiveness generally fades as fast as fireworks.

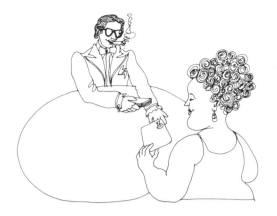

"The Cards Are Stacked against Me"

How a person eats, when he eats and how much he eats are all deeply rooted in the emotional history of the individual. Food is highly symbolic, according to psychologists, and it represents many different things to different people. But the most common denominator of such symbolism is that food means love. Madison Avenue knows it, and serves you "a little bit of love" along with many food advertisements. Madison Avenue knows your mother cuddled you, warmed you, and made you feel loved while you first learned the joys of eating, and it tries to convince you that their products will give you the same emotional security now. Advertisers know where you're vulnerable, so *you* might as well know it, too.

"Nobody loves me" is the feeling that drives most food-oriented people directly to the refrigerator, where love can be found in left-overs or cold cuts. Unfortunately, the obese person may have good reason to feel that "nobody loves me." Society today does not look with favor on the fat man, and it loves the fat woman even less. Certainly, drug addicts and alcoholics receive a more charitable reception and sympathetic treatment than does the food addict. The fat woman must add on an extra measure of obvious social disapproval for not being pleasant to behold. (Somehow, good looks are expected more of women than of men.) Self-dislike soon follows. In addition, our society holds that the fat person is not sexually attractive. Nor is he physically able to enjoy sex, if very heavy. As a result, food becomes an even more necessary comfort.

In teen-agers, who are breaking away from the family circle into their own identity anyway, the situation is especially painful if they are obese, and the need for love-substitutes more acute.

If the fat person becomes a patient, will the *doctor* love him? On the contrary, the obese patient is a source of frustration to doctor, psychologist, and researcher alike, a living failure. Top researchers tend to leave the field of obesity treatment because of the slow progress, the lack of government interest, and the apparent obstinacy of the fat condition.

When food is not a symbol of love, it may reflect hate. Resentment and hostility are sometimes expressed by overeating. Food can be involved in anger—just think of biting and chewing fiercely! A man relieves his anger at his dictatorial employer by eating a huge pacifying lunch. A teen-aged girl "gets even" with her preaching mother by eating half a cake. A bored wife finds comfort in sweets, and her added weight makes her unattractive to her husband; this punishes him for his failures and protects her from his sexual advances.

The dieter is well-advised to pamper himself a little, express a little self-love, associate with appreciative friends, dress as attractively as possible so as to approve of the person he sees in the mirror. He might give vent to his anger now and then, instead of expressing it in eating binges. A satisfactory sex life, of course, does help one to feel loved and therefore makes giving up other sensual treats that much easier. The more the feeling of being unloved or impotent against the tyrannical forces of life can be relieved in other ways than eating, the easier it will be to diet.

"A Barrel of Laughs..."

Thoughtful doctors readily admit that the obese are their most unhappy patients, thus dispelling the myth of the "jolly fat man."

The true measure of the desperation and depression of the obese is in the way they will grasp at any faint hope held out to them of improving their lot. They will "buy" health treatments like the "rainbow pills" at grave risk to their health, attempt punishing programs like fasting, or endure special surgery in order to reach a normal weight and a normal life. Surely, here we can detect motivation, fortitude, and determination. If only these helpful qualities would be channeled into equally helpful (but less dramatic) programs, much could be achieved.

Psychologists generally recognize the misery of the

obese, but they also find reasons in personal histories why this condition has occurred and how it supports certain "advantages" for the patient, such as defense against other anxieties.

Psychologists have also constructed "personality profiles" of the most common types of overeaters.

The first type, whom we will call Kurt Bigfellow, is an aggressive individual whose existence centers around oral activities. He not only eats great quantities of food with gusto, biting and tearing with zeal and even loudly sucking marrow from the bones, but, between meals, he can be found consuming large amounts of grog, chewing a cigar or pipe, and drowning out other conversation with his booming voice. Food, Kurt feels, makes him a "bigger" man and adds to his strength. If Kurt is attracted by real or imagined enemies or frustrated in his attempts to "get ahead," he will want to "build up" his "fortress" with even greater amounts of solid meat and potatoes.

Lily Languid, on the other hand, is a clinging vine, a passive and dependent gal to whom food offers warmth, love, and protection. Whenever Lily feels depressed and lonely, soft creamed foods and rich desserts give her comfort. Lily never gets angry at neglectful or abusive friends. Anger is present, of course, but she represses it because of her need for love.

Willie Shakeshoes is a timid soul whose desire is to insulate himself against "the slings and arrows of outrageous fortune" with a cushioning defense of fat. Anything which is bigger than he impresses Willie, and he eats in the hope of becoming equally impressive himself, at least in girth.

Gilda Gogetter has a high opinion of herself and

expects to be the constant center of attention. As a child, she was a tomboy, the leader of her gang, as a teenager, she was constantly dancing, bowling, skating, and so on. Marriage and the arrival of children slowed Gilda down considerably and also took her away from her circle of admiring friends. Feeding herself all the good food she deserved, as a substitute for excitement and attention, brought on a rapid weight gain. Gilda continues to enjoy special "treats" whenever she feels she lacks sufficient appreciation from her small family, and her "appetite" for this is a large one.

Rita Rebel lives in constant chaos, because organizing her life is too "establishment" for her. She's warm and friendly but fails to get along with people over a period of time due to her manipulations and demanding nature. She is impulsive and irresponsible, and, therefore, it is quite difficult for her to control her own eating habits. It is even more difficult for a doctor to put her on a diet, because Rita will fight against any kind of authority.

The motives ascribed to Kurt, Lily, Willie, Gilda, and Rita are, of course, *unconscious* ones. Consciously, all five of these people think they want to lose weight. They prefer to attempt the diets-doomed-to-failure rather than sensible methods, because of the psychological benefits when they fail. Nevertheless, they appear at diet clinics for help and advice—especially Lily and Willie. Lily likes advice for its own sake; it makes her feel loved. And Willie, who has no confidence in himself anyway, always feels that he needs the help of someone who is wiser. Kurt may be sent to a doctor by his company, which is interested in his health; Gilda may look for attention from the medical profession when other alternatives fail; and Rita wants someone else to get her organized, although later she will defy all advice.

These are caricatures, of course, but it profits the dieter to become aware of what foods and fatness may represent to him in the way of unconscious benefits. When he feels his good resolves weakening, he can try to provide appropriate substitutes instead of eating more. If Lily is downcast over the loss of a friend, for example, she could seek out the company of another friend rather than stay at home and eat a quart of pistachio ice cream.

The problem with surrendering to a temporary psychological need for rich, fattening foods is that your appestat setting may be raised higher during the process. Later, when problems have been solved and anxieties abate, the setting remains high and your appetite continues to call for excessive food intake. Going back on your diet will involve another real battle with honest hunger.

There may be times when a doctor would best serve the health needs of his obese patient by taking into account psychological requirements and not making unrealistic demands for weight reduction. Obesity may be due to the need to overeat or the need to *be* overweight—or both! A judgement should be made about the patient's ability to tolerate weight loss psychologically. This means it would be better to go to your regular physician, who at least knows something about you and your history, rather than an unknown and unknowing "diet doctor."

Patience and persistence are your most helpful attributes in dieting to lose weight. Patience helps in realizing the importance of taking your time—no seven days to a marvelous new figure and a nervous breakdown, please! Persistence is needed when you reach a stage where for two weeks you don't lose an ounce no matter how you wiggle the scale. This is called a "plateau," and it happens to the best of dieters. The idea is just to keep on with your healthful, slimming meals. At least, you know they're *good* for you, even if you're not losing weight at that very moment. Eventually you will begin to lose again.

Dr. Henry A. Jordan, of University of Pennsylvania Medical School, is working on the problem of long-term obesity. "Once they (the obese) stay at a given weight for a long period of time, that becomes a new equilibrium for them," he declares, and it is his hope that new ways will be found to uncover the key to the equilibrium mystery and a solution to the problem of excess fat cells.

These findings emphasize the necessity of getting at a weight problem in its early stages, rather than permitting a gain of twenty pounds to persist for years. The longer you are overweight, the more difficult the weight will be to lose as you begin the struggle to change what has become a new weight equilibrium for you. But, even the loss of *part* of your overweight is better than no loss at all!

Another unhappy conclusion physicians have reached is that obesity is seldom cured, taking into account the metabolic and the psychological factors involved. If, however, obesity is to be successfully treated, it must be emphasized to the patient that he will be "on a diet" for the rest of his life. We only wish there were some other phrase, because "diet" is another one of those words with an uninviting reputation, like "habit." So let us quickly add that we don't mean a *semi-starvation diet,* but a "life diet" of new, more healthful, less fattening foods. Otherwise, one will merely regain the lost weight as soon as the old eating habits that got one into an overweight condition in the first place are reinstated.

Dr. Neil Solomon seems to have coined the phrase "yo-yo syndrome" to describe the cyclical losing and regaining of weight that many obese persons go through, especially when metabolic abnormalities exist. He believes, however, that these abnormalities may be the *result* rather than the *cause* of overweight, and the right diet can make it possible not only to lose weight but to "stabilize" weight also—in other words, to kick the "yo-yo syndrome" forever!

The key phrase there is "the right diet." Every doctor with a book in print (and there are many!) has a different idea about what constitutes this magic formula, and it is the problem of the dieter to sort through this avalanche of menus and counting tables and warnings and assurances to come up with the diet which will work for him personally.

If (for example) a dieter who has high blood pressure follows the invitation to enjoy all the meat and cheese he can eat on a low-carbohydrate diet, he has to limit himself on the salty salami and hard cheeses, because salt can be dangerous to him. One man's luncheon meat is another man's poison! Someone with a tricky digestion is going to run into trouble with "all the fats, butter, mayonnaise, and cream that you want," unless he uses a measure of caution.

What we hope to do in this book is to present

finally the conclusions on which *most* authorities agree, theories for which there is an *adequate* amount of supportive scientific evidence. For example, it has been clearly shown by *many* experiments that the carbohydrate level in a diet must be kept low if a person is going to lose weight. There is also excellent evidence to support the body's ability to restore itself to normality metabolically when fat is lost.

The fat person may be "the life of the party" in public, but, in private, if he wants to lose weight, he is probably burning the midnight oil to read diet book after diet book, compare grams to calories, weigh fruit diets against meat diets, weigh *himself* every half hour, and worry whether the grapefruit he had for breakfast is really going to help "dissolve" his fat or has completely upset his "carbo-cal" count for the day. In short, he's a very troubled soul, who well may cry, "O! That this too, too solid flesh might melt . . ."

A Rousing Cheer for Change

In a popular book on psychology called *I'm OK— You're OK,* Dr. Thomas A. Harris has a very hopeful message for those who want to alter the destructive habits of the past; he believes in a person's ability to change. Since much of the medical literature we've been quoting has provided the reader with sobering statistics on the difficulties of treating obesity, it's refreshing to find someone putting faith in the future as well as recognizing the importance of the past.

Dr. Harris describes three conditions which he says make people *want* to change. First, they have to "hurt sufficiently," and, in the case of the obese, that would be how a fat person feels when he really allows himself to recognize the limitations that overweight places on all areas of his life—those limitations do "hurt"! Secondly, Dr. Harris points to an *ennui* or boredom with the present state of affairs that reaches the proportions of despair. Thirdly, people *want* to change when they discover that they *can* change. Self-causation is as much of a force as outside causes on the life of an individual.

Although he recognizes the strength of past conditioning, Dr. Harris is still putting all his chips on "free will," and he reminds us that Ortega defines man as "a being which consists not so much in what it is as in what it is going to be."

Discoveries and theories about the psychological factors which influence obesity show an undeniable connection between emotions and eating habits, but this is only a part of the picture, as the physical description of obesity is only a part, also. But we subscribe to the theory that, no matter how many times a man (and a dieter) may have failed, the possibility of success is still very real and worth working to attain.

Play To Block "Future Fat"

From man's beginnings on this planet until very recently, he has had to struggle to get enough food to stay alive. Yet, almost overnight, it has become essential to "shift gears," to reverse our instinctive attitude that the more we eat the healthier we are. Overweight is no longer the status symbol it once was. Today it has become, instead, "Public Enemy Number One."

Overweight people tend to die at an earlier age than people of normal weight; therefore, it is a matter of serious social concern.

Most doctors are in agreement as to the dangers of obesity, and insurance companies reinforce this conviction with their mortality statistics. Some authorities even state that obesity is associated with all leading causes of death today. But so much still remains to be discovered and understood about this subject that it isn't at all clear when obesity is the cause of a disease, when it is the result of a disease, and when it is in coincidence with a disease. A great deal of research still needs to be done.

Not that there aren't some dissenting views. One Columbia psychiatrist, Hilde Bruch, is quoted as saying, "I have come to the conclusion that it is basically wrong and leads to a biased misinterpretation of the whole problem to start with the prior assumption that overweight is invariably harmful and an unmitigated evil, without any possible value for the carrier . . ." Bruch suggests that one obstacle to a "more meaningful and rational approach to the whole obesity problem" is the present-day attitude which considers the slightest sign of rounded contours as "ugly signs of greedy self-indulgence."

The changes in social awareness and health consciousness have also affected changes in statistics on dieting. During the "Roaring Twenties," fashions became more daring and women became more conscious of their newly-revealed figures. During the Fifties, twice as many women as men were still concerned with those extra pounds, and one woman out of three had tried to lose weight, as opposed to one man out of seven. But, in the Sixties, some men, at least, were beginning to heed the warnings about the possible connection between overweight and heart disease.

Research polls showed that men dieted longer and lost somewhat more per diet than women, almost 14 pounds as against about 12½ for the women. Of the men polled, 66 percent said they dieted for reasons of health rather than looks. The average for health dieters among the females was 48 percent. Vanity, however, is still apparently a stronger motive for dieting than the fear of early death. Although the country's weight average for women has been on a steady decline since the Twenties, the weight average for men has been going up. And women still outnumber men in attempting to diet, 72 percent compared to 28 percent. Among the clinically obese, however—those who are 20 percent or more above their ideal weight—the women outnumber the men three to two (21,000,000 to 14,000,-000). Obviously, the women "try harder," but they seem to be less successful dieters.

Why is it so difficult? Most often, people have a problem in sticking to a diet regimen. The average dieter goes on one and a quarter diets per year, and "cutting down" sometimes involves little more than using an artificial sweetener in coffee or a "diet" soft drink instead of a regular "cola." Even those who attempt a "diet plan" have not shown encouraging results. The average "diet" lasts only between 60 and 90 days, and, during that period, the dieter is apt to "cheat" for about half the time. There may be "honor among thieves," but dieters are another matter!

Obviously, the "diets," whether obtained from popular magazines or professional sources, are inadequate in meeting all the "satisfaction demands" of the individual. Perhaps those who are overweight need to begin to think in terms of a whole set of new eating habits, rather than a short-term "punishment" diet for having raided the cookie jar too often.

Bootleg Beefburgers, Anyone?

Peter Wyden, in his book *The Overweight Society,* says that the "abundance of food must eventually lead to social controls on calories." He asks the question, "How many people will die needlessly before we begin to construct these controls?"

Wyden has an interesting solution on which to speculate. For a first step, he suggests making readily available "the best facts and counsel" to the public. This information would be generated from "the best experts, under Presidential sponsorship," who would interrupt their fragmented pursuits of the problem to "discuss all of its elements at the summit level, and then issue at least a progress report to demolish unnecessary public uncertainties." He suggests that "parents, physicians, educators, researchers, industrial interests, and the government guardians over our health and food" work together in a concerted assault on the overweight problem.

This is obviously a well-meaning proposal, and, just as obviously, there are a lot of unanswered questions in it. Not only is the thought of any additional "controls" in our society repugnant to many people, but the effectiveness of such controls is very uncertain. Secondly, which "experts" shall be invited to the "summit level" conferences? Experts are available who will support every tenuous theory and who will contradict the theories of other experts. And how will the emphasis be shifted from immediate profit to national well-being in "industrial interests?" Government officials, who are generally a well-fed-looking lot, might better concentrate on slimming down the Senate before they branch out to counsel on weight welfare to the nation.

Fascinating as this is in conjecture, the problem, as is true of most problems, should be "reduced" to its most realistic proportions. The individual is the one who must finally take the responsibility for change in himself. Enough individuals assuming the proper "control" of their own eating habits can bring about the desired national change. Information on good health and diet must be provided, of course, but the rest is up to the dieter. He, after all, is alone with his refrigerator at midnight and must make all the final decisions.

Future Fat

Obesity is a matter for social concern, and the implications of the problem on a national scale are reminiscent of the fate of the ancient Romans. Their life-style led, eventually, to a very bad time when those hardy, lean Huns descended on the fat, soft citizens of Rome—a city where Lucullan feasts were the order of the day. According to Peter Wyden, doctors of our time are accepting the fact that obesity is an important social problem "whose solution is non-existent."

Wyden quotes Dr. Philip L. White, Director of the American Medical Association's Department of Foods and Nutrition, as telling him privately, "I'm inclined to say, 'Let's let the present generation go ahead and wallow in its fat and worry about the young people'."

But the problem, from a national standpoint, can no more be ignored for a generation than can an epidemic of major proportions. The desirable solution, of course, would be the prevention of obesity. Dr. Jean Mayer, of Harvard, has said, "If there's one disease condition where an ounce of prevention is better than a pound of cure, it is obesity."

If one is already pretty hefty, these words do become a bit of hindsight rhetoric. Yet, this is a goal we can all work toward in the case of children and, especially, very young children and infants. Common sense in feeding children and babies, encouraging healthful eating habits, and discouraging reliance early in life on "empty calories" as short-cut meals would be excellent first steps in the right direction.

In his book, *The Fight Against Obesity,* Dr. Roger Williams warns that "no deficiencies should be allowed to perpetuate themselves." The feeding of obesity-prone children requires the same attention as the feeding of babies susceptible to any other disease. "Certainly the use of naked calories—particularly sugar—should be discouraged," Dr. Williams goes on to say. Nutritional deficiency leads to "sugar hunger," and "a vicious cycle is thus established. Poor nutrition fosters worse nutrition." In the young, proper brain development, among other things, depends rather heavily on good nutrition.

Proper nutrition for children becomes even more important when one realizes that, once a person has been obese, some irreversible physiologic changes occur which, according to Dr. Mayer, may make the regaining of weight previously lost more "efficient" than the original weight gain. It is essential that pediatricians and school physicians be made aware of the necessity for an intelligent program of diet and exercise for the obesity-prone youngsters in their care.

In a study of six hungry volunteers, aged 11 to 15, conducted in Mexico a few years ago, the youngsters were tested before and after being shown appetizing meals which they were not permitted to eat. Within 20 minutes of seeing the food, there was a marked chemical change in their systems which indicated that external stimuli are just as powerful for the young as for the old.

Parents themselves are often the agents of potential danger for obesity-prone children. The mother who tries to quiet her crying baby with a cookie or the grandparent who insures receiving affection from a child by favoring the young one with candy are hardly the "best friends" a kid can have. Along with other future difficulties, such "loving care" may be starting the child along the path to obesity.

The tubby tot is excluded from games and play by his thinner, more active peers—and his own embarrassed sense of inadequacy and awkwardness can make him almost a recluse. It's tough enough for an adult who can intellectually grasp the reasons for his situation. The youngster can only feel hurt and bewildered. He is told he will "outgrow his baby fat," but this is not automatically true.

Leading authorities are finding that just being fat is a serious threat to children both physically and emotionally, and experts are genuinely alarmed at the enormous number of overweight children in our society. Nation-wide, more than 10,000,000 young people below the age of nineteen are overweight. Dr. J. T. Keeve, administrator of the school health program of Newburg, New York, said, in *The Journal of School*

Health, "A chief reason for concern is the fact that juvenile obesity not only persists into adult life but tends to be more severe and more difficult to treat than obesity occurring in adult life."

The beaming mother who brags about how much her baby eats strikes envy into the heart of the mother whose baby seems satisfied with just his formula. This envious mother badgers the pediatrician until he prescribes some solid food for her baby, too. Dr. Richard G. Goldbloom, Physician in Chief for the Children's Hospital of Halifax, Nova Scotia, says, "In recent years there has been a competitive spirit abroad in North America. Mothers often vie with each other to see who can introduce her infant to the most foods at the earliest possible moment of life." Rapid weight gain, he suggests, is not equivalent to robust health "in infancy any more than it is in later years of life."

Doctors and medical people are also contributors to the problem of obesity in children. Dr. J. J. Oldfield of Thirsk, Yorkshire, writing in *The British Medical Journal,* is dismayed to hear visiting and public health personnel advising young mothers to "start supplementary fat-making carbohydrate feeding from the early age of three or four weeks, whether the baby be breast- or bottle-fed." According to Dr. Oldfield, it's high time for a complete revision of baby, infant, and child dietetics to promote the development of a thinner, healthier adult, rather than "laying down an unhealthy feeding pattern for life."

One half of all fat children are seriously overweight by their sixth birthdays. Obesity in childhood is linked to hyperinsulin, according to an item in *Modern Medicine* quoting Drs. Malcom M. Martin and

Arline I. A. Martin. "With increasing age and duration of obesity, there is a definite tendency for lasting insulin concentrations to rise, insulin response to glucose to increase, and carbohydrate tolerance to deteriorate in obese children. Chemical diabetes is more prevalent among older obese children than published data indicate, possibly because of prolonged overweight or sex hormone secretion, or both."

Parents can help the potentially obese child by encouraging enjoyable activities—sports, games, walks —especially if the child shows a tendency to be sedentary. A fat child should never be shamed by his parents through the use of unflattering nicknames. Both parents can provide the child with a tactful, understanding, warm, and supportive atmosphere, so that he will not be so quick to seek solace in "sweet" calories.

Doctors and psychologists who have treated obesity in children, often teen-agers, find that the children are more likely to keep to a new eating regimen if the parents refrain from comment. If, however, in an effort to "help" the program, there is nagging in the home over every morsel the youngster puts into his mouth, the diet is almost certain to be abandoned. Once the problem has reached the stage where medical help is sought, parents can help by providing the right foods, eliminating the tempting snacks, and allowing the young person to develop his own program with the assistance of the medical advisor.

Children represent the future of our society. We adults are charged with the responsibility of preparing them for that future. It will avail society very little if its citizens are unable to function meaningfully because their physical condition makes it difficult for them to move about. It will not be enough that we have done our utmost to insure that they receive a proper education. Our children also need healthy vigorous bodies with which to enjoy the fruits of education.

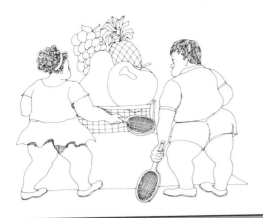

If You're Not Winning, Switch Courts

Even with the help of science fiction, no one knows exactly how the further development of automation is going to affect society. Certain aspects are clear, however. The use of automated systems and machines will increase rather than decrease. In order to lessen employment problems, unions will succeed in reducing the work week drastically. The amount and variety of goods, including exotic food items, available to the consumer will increase as automation is improved and streamlined. Relieved of the more routine and tedious tasks, people will find themselves with an excess of leisure time on their hands. Isn't that a wonderful picture, a fabulous and luxurious future to which we can all look forward! Just one serpent in the Garden of Eden, though. Less work and more eating makes Jack a fat cat!

Obviously, the individual is going to have to find ways to keep fit—to use up energy, pleasurably, in this brave, new world and, if not to eat less exactly, to eat *better!* Leisure will be that much more enjoyable and zesty if it includes active sports and games. If one cannot change the trend of social development, one must compensate with a life style that will enable him to function actively in the world, rather than fall into a stupor for hours in front of the TV. Even reading, which may be fine for broadening the mind, needs to be relieved by some form of physical romp, to avoid broadening the bottom as well.

But life, with all its technological "helpers" and gadgets becomes so "comfortable," it's difficult to make one's self leap out of a chair for a fast game when someone cries "tennis, anyone?" To some it may appear an eccentricity bordering on the Spartan to refuse to fall victim to such pleasant ease, offered so enticingly by leisure. But it is necessary. We assume that those "government controls" suggested by Wyden are not going to come about, and it will be up to each individual to maintain his fitness of body.

In his book, *The Overweight Society,* Wyden did provide us with some alarming statistics. For instance, potato chips sales in 1951 grossed $243,630,000. By 1962, they had risen to $580,780,000. At 10 calories and 35 percent fat per chip, that's a lot of potential poundage, especially when you take into consideration the usual location of the potato chip bowl—right beside the easy chair! Judging by the space afforded to this "goodie" in supermarkets and the ever-increasing giant-to-mammoth size of those shiny plastic bags, potato chip sales for this year will surely be much higher.

And that's only *one* part of a panorama of snack foods our society has accepted without thought or question.

How do we get all those potato chips home? Wheels to the supermarket, wheels through the aisle and to the check-out counter, and wheels home. Or, if you really want to do it in style, reach for the phone and have them delivered! This could be called "The Great Potato Chip Plot," engineered by merchandising *banditos* who only want to make a profit. The Romans had a phrase that covers the situation—*caveat emptor* (let the buyer beware).

In the A.M.A. Journal for January 10, 1966, Ashley Montagu, in his article "Obesity and the Evolution of Man," says, "Obesity cannot have been an advantage at any time in the evolution of man." For berry-pickers and hunters of paleolithic times to eat to the point of obesity, even if such a supply was occasionally available, would have severely interfered with their capacity of foraging for food.

The establishment of farming and city environments was the initiator of obesity, at least for the wealthier segments of the population. In many societies, obesity became recognized as a status symbol. If a man were fat, if his wife or wives were fat, if his children were fat, if his cattle were fat, and if even his servants were chubby, it meant he was rich enough to provide abundantly. "In many communities," says Dr. Montagu, "being well-padded came to stand not only for affluence but also for the ability to survive." This may explain why so many mothers in our society still worry about their children if they're not plump and rosy. "A custom originating in earlier more stressful times," adds Dr. Montagu, which "has continued into the present where it no longer serves a useful purpose."

"But I Made It Just for You!"

How easily does one shake off the influences of a cultural heritage where rich, fattening foods were not only a part of the physical life but were also intrinsically bound to the social life as well? We're all familiar with the image of the ethnic mother, opulently rounded herself, whose idea of a "small" piece of cake is any slice that's smaller than a breadbox. There are the homes in which holiday meals least three or four hours, and each course would be sufficient for a full meal, but each is followed by another, even more impressive and tempting. On such occasions hard-working people got together and relaxed, cracked jokes, drank, laughed, and ate—and ate and ate! The custom continues today in many areas. The question is, how much can we blame these cultural and environmental influences for our present struggle with overweight.

It may be that this is not as important a factor as we have believed. Evidently, attempts by youngsters to move outside the "Establishment" have succeeded sufficiently to make obesity more of a random occurrence than an ethnic outgrowth. In a paper on genetics in obesity, published in *Postgraduate Medicine,* April, 1965, Harvard's Jean Mayer mentions research conducted on the influence and effect of cultural backgrounds interacting with genetics in the overweight problem. He reports on a study conducted by J. L. Angel: in a large group of obese persons surveyed, 42.7 percent had American-born parents, 8.7 percent were American-born of foreign-born parents, and

13.6 percent were foreign-born. Claims have been made (on the basis of limited samples) concerning the high incidence of obesity "among children of South European and Jewish stock," but further studies simply have not confirmed this theory.

So if you've been blaming your overweight problem on pizza or knishes stuffed into your mouth by a dutiful mama, it may be illuminating to realize that many of your compatriots have come out of the very same backgrounds without an extra ounce of flab on their bones. (Although somewhere there may be mothers who consider themselves failures because of it.)

"Nothin' Says Lovin' Like Something from the Oven" and Other Misconceptions

Unfortunately, the overweight person is the frequent butt of jokes and scorn, especially during adolescence, when a chorus of "I don't want her, you can have her, she's too fat for me," can become a major tragedy to the one who is thus serenaded. The discriminations and recriminations continue into adult life. Fashion designers concern themselves with a size eight figure; the plump young woman has a frustrating time of it buying clothes and may very well end up with an outfit that looks as if it were designed for the mother of a bride.

Insurance premiums are higher for obese people. Family, "friends," doctors, and the advertising media are constantly pointing out that extra pounds are ugly, out of fashion, and the sure sign of a spineless character with no will power. One would assume from this that the obese constitute a minority, easy to torment and castigate. Yet we have seen what the statistics reveal. One wonders if those who are pointing the finger of scorn have been looking in the mirror.

While the obese person is truly and unjustifiably a victim of social bias, the gravest injustice of all is how easily he is exploited by the advertising paid for by profit-hungry industries. First he falls victim to the lure of the succulent food commercials. Then, anxious for remedies, he falls prey to cleverly-worded promises of immediate results in diet foods, diet drugs, and exercise equipment that is at best useless and at worst harmful.

The advertising media's job is to sell—through suggestion, cajoling, innuendo, and, if that fails, outright insult and scolding. Improbable and fantastic claims are made for the touted products in language just this side of possible prosecution for fraud. (Now and then, some company slips over the line there, and sometimes an alert government agency gets them!)

Picking the pocket of obese America seems to be as easy as picking corn at harvest-time. On the one hand, we are bombarded by the TV with "instant and piping hot," "just like home made," "melt-in-your-mouth," "drenched-in-butter-sauce" vegetables and meats, cooked especially for you by folks as warm and nice as your own Ma. On the other hand, we have a mature, sincere, white-coated father figure, who looks as much like Marcus Welby as possible, offering you the fastest antacid in the West. This is followed by a lovely young lady, so slim that the camera has to shoot her in long, lingering sections while she draws one tapering ectomorphic finger down a pyramid of diet drink bottles with only a fraction of a calorie per case (the rest is chemicals).

If you turn off the TV to read a magazine, turn to the "food" section and you'll find at least half a hundred recipes for dishes that you can make for under ten dollars and over a thousand calories. If it's the Christmas issue, you get more recipes and the plans for constructing a life-size gingerbread house for the kids to eat before they go back to school after New Year's Day. These easy-to-prepare recipes (easy if you are a graduate of the *Cordon Bleu*) are cleverly dovetailed with full-color, full-page advertisements of products you use to make these dishes.

Then, under "Beauty," you'll find the latest so-you're-going-to-The-Company-Party-on-Saturday-and-nothing-fits 5-day reducing diet. And, as you reach the back of the magazine, advertisements will offer you sure-fire bust developers, hip and thigh reducing shorts that look like hot pants for a hippopotamus, diet "candy" endorsed by stars of stage, screen, and radio, and exercise equipment that requires no more effort than reaching into your pocket for the money to pay for it.

People are impatient. They want instant results, easy "cures," and so they let themselves be victimized again and again. Advertisers are not on the side of the consumer; it's their clients who pay their salaries.

Don't be misled by "testimonials" or articles by doctors calling themselves "obesity specialists." Not all of their remedies are safe, healthful, or suited to you personally. Wyden mentions "obesity specialists who sometimes use research and professional journals to legitimatize alleged weight-reducing products . . ."

Irving Ladimer, a vice president of the National Better Business Bureau, has listed types of obesity-research specialists that both public and medical men should be wary of: the "Professional Investigator," always ready to undertake a study for anyone who asks him, whether or not he is qualified to do the study; the "House Doctor," who produces the "right" results in his tests; and certain products whose efficacy is backed by medical investigations "conducted by men who have been granted stock options in the manufacturing house." Ladimer indicates that, because of these situations, "some medical journals have thus become 'inadvertent co-promoters of quackery.' "

The pitfalls are many, and the nonsense is thick in the air. There are no instant, magic shortcuts. But there are things you can do for yourself. You'll protect yourself from the exploiters if you develop a life style that assures you a healthy body at a sensible weight. That's what this book is all about.

Getting It All Together

Surely people as ingenious as ours, who have faced so many crises and mastered them, can find a way to cope with any national problem, including obesity. "The American Way," of course, is to organize— and we see the first faint glimmers of organization beginning to "zero in" on the broad target that obesity presents. In lieu of government action, we have a spate of diet clubs like Weight Watchers and TOPS, a new medical specialty "Bariatrics" (treatment of the obese), and the National Association to Aid Fat Americans or

NAAFA. These groups have proved helpful to many people, each in its own way.

Hopefully, the American Society of Bariatrics will work toward a more responsible handling of obese patients than we have seen in the past decade, when some doctors made a fortune handing out "rainbow pills" until a few people died from that rigorous combination of drugs. Dr. Ervin Barr, a bariatrician, laments the fact that a great many doctors "pretend knowledge" of obesity cures and hand out appetite-depressant pills too readily. He says it is these doctors who give his speciality a "quack" reputation.

According to Dr. Barr, there are only about 300 doctors who are actually members of the American Society of Bariatrics. "It is extremely important," adds Dr. Barr, "when you're advising an obese individual that you treat the whole person—not an appendage called fat." He feels that counting calories is not the answer. "Measuring what you eat," he points out, "is a great way to take the joy out of life—but not to take off pounds or inches!" Nor does he believe that solutions lie in the adherence to strange diets that advocate special concentration on certain foods (like bananas or grapefruit) as though the consumption of these foods to the degree advised would work a chemical miracle in the body and melt the fat away.

The diet clubs have accumulated a substantial number of avid adherents and they continue to attract new members. In fact, they are on their way to becoming a big business, as diversification leads them into producing their own brand of frozen dinners and other specialties. Certainly, an awesome amount of poundage has been lost, and, for people who find the group situation a supportive one, the clubs have a great deal to offer.

Inspiring speakers and catchy tunes make it a pleasant social occasion, and the no-sugar, very-low-fat, low-carbohydrate, high-protein diets they feature keep people feeling peppy while they lose weight—especially those who have never eaten a real breakfast, as they are forced to do on this regimen. Unfortunately, their efforts to give their members substitute desserts encourage the use of a number of undesirable chemical "sweets," and the kind of bread they permit is about as nutritious and tasty as library paste.

Taking a lesson from the highly effective example of Alcoholics Anonymous, these clubs use much of the same psychology. Like A.A., they also tend to promote dependent "life members" who keep attending meetings after they have achieved their weight goals, in an effort to prevent backsliding. A "penalty"—a charge for attending that evening's meeting—is imposed on those "graduates" present who have gained three pounds or more *over* that ideal figure. (There might be enough salt in a salami sandwich and a "side" of potato chips to retain three pounds of fluid. Such carelessness in food selection by the member results in an extra source of revenue for the club.)

NAAFA's efforts, as previously explained, are not in the direction of changing the condition of obesity but rather to provide a happier environment for the overweight segment of the population through social improvement. You don't have to be fat to join; you only have to send $10.00 (or $15.00 if you live in a foreign country). According to their brochure, "fat people sometimes have trouble merely being treated like human beings who have the same needs and rights as everybody else!" Their stated aim is to attack "the problem from all possible angles; we are continually seeking new ways to help our members (and others) find dignity and happiness in their lives." They disseminate a newsletter to members and frequently engage in letter-writing campaigns to combat job discrimination against overweight people, and to try to influence advertising agencies and the clothing industry to admit that people who aren't built like Twiggy, and never will be, also need clothes.

Whether the emphasis is on helping the problem of obesity or on companionable cameraderie, group efforts continue to thrive, and "fat power" is beginning to make itself felt.

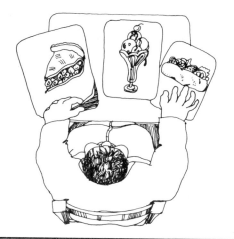

Solitaire—Don't Cheat the Dealer

The reasons why one person is fat generally have little similarity to the reasons why another person is fat. It isn't so much that the body processes themselves are different from one person to the next. It's the intricate combination of physical causes acting in relation to the psychological influences of personal history, plus the social pressures experienced by the individual. Each of these factors plays a role in the drama of the body's functioning that makes each case of obesity truly unique.

Attempting to treat a person with a weight problem according to standard formulas only leads to further frustration in most cases. The entire personality as well as the state of physical being must be taken into account, along with attitudes toward and interaction with social environment. Treatment should be guided by a cognizance of all influences as they relate *to a particular case.*

"What is good for one person may be absolutely worthless to another," says University of Pennsylvania Medical School's Dr. Henry A. Jordan. He adds that "each person carries a different combination of genetic, psychological and behavioral problems." Treating them "across the board" will, he believes, only lead to "the same hit-or-miss approach that has characterized the treatment of obesity in the past."

We know that few overweight persons can be satisfactorily helped by any generalized method emanating from "instant-result" prescriptions, drug company "discoveries," or a ghost-written doctor's theory. Does that mean that every individual must seek an extensive and expensive personal regimen from experts in all fields? No—it means that he has to get to know himself—his strengths and weaknesses, even his peccadillos and prejudices—well enough to adapt the best of current knowledge on the subject to his own unique life-style.

Consider a very broad example of differences in life-style: some people eat lunch at home every day and some "brown bag" it, but some are forced to lunch in restaurants. Any diet such a person chooses will have to be adapted to the realities of his day-to-day temptations.

In the final analysis, most people are going to have to work out their own salvation. Experts are able to offer "guides," encouragement, motivation, and a wealth of case histories for interesting reading. They can lead a dieter to the table, but they can't put the right foods in his mouth.

Dr. Howard D. Kurland, Chief of the Psychiatry Service at the Veterans Administration Research Hospital and Assistant Professor at the Northwestern University Medical School, believes that the extremely obese individual seeks to change his relationship with the world by becoming fat. The "psychologic effects of massive adiposity" are his "protection." Dr. Kurland makes a comparison with the drug addict whose need is not to swallow or jab the drug into his system but to alter his state of consciousness in order to alter his relationship with the world around him. In the case of food addicts, the point is made that the person may not need to eat a lot as much as to weigh a lot. Once off a diet, he will seek to regain his lost "buffer," his protection of fat, and the restrictions of physical, social, and sexual activities that accompany obesity.

If this were the only motivation at work in the individual, he would not, of course, go on a diet in the first place, or even read a book like this one. However, many times the fat person does consciously want to lose weight and is unable to deal with unconscious motivations to remain fat, especially if he is unaware of them. You wouldn't be able to get a car to run, either, if you had a leak in the transmission and were unaware of it. One half of the battle is self-knowledge and motivation; the other half is accurate and responsible advice.

Many desperate overweight people have tried fasting or have, at least, considered it. This is a good example of when responsible advice and accurate information are needed. Dr. George Edward Schauf, in a paper published in the August 1973 issue of the *Journal of the American Geriatric Society,* offered an interesting explanation of the formation of fat and the effects of fasting on the body. Certain body elements—the brain, nervous system, adrenal medulla, germinal layers of the gonads, and erythrocyles during glycolysis only—are obligatory users of glucose. The muscles, kidney, heart, and liver (the main lean-mass tissues) "use free fatty acid as a primary energy," Dr. Schauf writes. He described stored glycogen in the muscles (used mainly in states of oxygen debt) and ketone bodies formed in the liver "during glycogen depletion states from the partial oxidation of fatty acids, as secondary energy sources." Extended periods of starvation bring about the oxidation of ketones by the lean tissues, and, Dr. Schauf believes, to some extent by the brain.

According to Dr. Schauf, when the individual is storing fat in his fat cells, he's becoming obese (and this is the generally accepted definition of obesity), but when fatty acids leave the fat cells and are oxidized by the muscles and other lean tissues "obesity is diminished." Improper diets or brief periods of starvation will result in weight loss but not necessarily in fat loss. Dr. Schauf reports on recent experiments which demonstrated that subjects who ate no food at all for from 10 to 17 days, lost weight. But 59 to 66 percent of the loss was a contribution of lean tissues. "Since lean tissues oxidize free fatty acid as a primary energy, dietary regimens which cause loss of lean tissue will proportionately decrease the body's capacity to oxidize and lose fat."

Lean tissue, of course, is not what an obese person wants to lose. He wants to be rid of the layers of fat crowded in those fat cells. His diet must be designed to reduce fat while sparing lean tissue, so that he will remain healthy while reducing.

Fasting, then, actually delays the "cure" of obesity, although it does bring about a temporary weight loss. Yet fasting has been tried under hospital conditions, and even sanctioned by private doctors for patients dieting at home.

Carbohydrates are again cited as promoters of fat formation, but many diets, especially "low-calorie" diets, do not make any distinction between what kind of calories you are consuming—yet, as you can see, it makes quite a difference to the body.

Exercise not only helps to "burn up" energy and increases muscle tone (which keeps you looking good while you lose weight), but actually helps the body to oxidize fatty acid. This brings us back to the influence of social factors in obesity. Ever try to walk a mile on a Sunday to pick up the papers? Chances are some well-meaning neighbor will stop and offer you a ride, assuming that something must have happened to your car. Ever try to mow your lawn with an unpowered mower? Someone will lend you a powered one that you may even be able to sit on intead of walking behind it. Children are driven to school, whereupon some of their class time has to be spent in physical exercise to keep fit, while the "free" exercise of walking to school is scorned.

As we have said, each case has its own unique ramifications, and it may be that one person has a great deal of difficulty in just finding the time in which to exercise, while another has time but has just gotten into a pattern of sedentary habits. There are differences in abilities and preferences to consider. The exercise program that will fit you best will be the one which you yourself develop to fit your personality and your life, although you may have to be a bit Machiavellian to carry it out in our society.

On Leading a Life of Diet Desperation

The problem of obesity affects more people, engenders more theories, offers more fads, and makes more hucksters extremely wealthy, while evoking less understanding and compassion for the victim, than any other single medical condition.

In the midst of serious and well-intentioned research into the subject of obesity, in the chaos of contradicting theories surrounding the problem, lies another complication for the desperate dieter—fraud! The element of fraud, or "huckstering," is not only heartless but, at times, tragic for the victim. Both in and out of the medical profession, there are "sharpies" and "quacks" ready to prey on the lean pocketbooks of the fat dieters.

No medical problem has a greater number of "experts" nor a smaller number of "cures" than obesity—and this one fact in itself should be a tip off that charlatans are at work. Profiteers, having discovered that there is money to be made in this lucrative field, have been barraging the market with fantastic diets and miracle slenderizers.

No other physical condition arouses so many guilt feelings in the victim as obesity does. Along with physical and emotional problems, in addition to social pressures and peer disapproval with which a fat person must contend, he must also be alert (to the point of being suspicious) concerning those anxious to "help" him. He must learn to distinguish between genuine offers of help and offers by those who intend to "help themselves" to his savings. This is an added burden that the obese person certainly doesn't need!

Shelves in the drugstore and the supermarket are filled with "answers" to the fat person's prayers. But which one is the right answer? The more desperate the dieter becomes, the more alternatives he will probably try during the course of his "battle of the bulge." Doctors have warned again and again that any remedy strong enough to have some measurable effect will only be available by prescription, and remedies available in the stores without a prescription are too weak to accomplish all they claim. (Any weight loss they achieve will be due to the accompanying "diet plan" hidden inside the package.)

Consulting with a physician is another solution for the dieter. Hopefully, the doctor will do more than pass along a Xeroxed 1,000 calorie-a-day diet and a pat on the back. If the patient is lucky, he will get a complete examination and the physician will not be at work on a pet theory of his own so that the patient becomes another experiment in the doctor's laboratory. It will also better serve the purposes of the patient if the physician has no professional connection with any drug manufacturer or distributor. These are a lot of "if's"— which is not to discount the sincere work being done by many responsible medical men in this difficult field.

The road an obese person travels is often lonely—

and, unfortunately, full of these pesky potholes. Your physician may prescribe drugs and your psychiatrist may lend you his ear and his couch (although, you'd be better off if you'd pace up and down while talking to him)—but you are the one who will finally have to remedy the problem. The right road will be an uphill one, but not unsafe or unpleasant. It will lead, through wise nutrition and sensible exercise, to healthful reducing regimens—and it will lead there *every* time!

What can you do to protect yourself against frauds, fads, and quacks? If you have an overweight problem, be realistic about it—and be realistic, too, about the world around you. The problem grew slowly, and it will be cured slowly. It will always take some effort on your part, no solution will be effortless or miraculous.

In *The Overweight Society,* Wyden takes a Disneyland-like trip through a place he calls "Dietland," which is sub-divided into "semi-autonomous principalities." In "Expertland," a great debate wages between doctors, psychologists, nutritionists, and motivational researchers. In "Groanerland," those rotund tummies are being flattened by exercise in health spas. In "Playland," expensive reducing resorts are supplemented with "low-cost group-therapy classes where students are invited to embarrass each other into taking off poundage." In "Quackland," pills and gadgets and fad diets abound. "Profitland" is the home of conflicting books about calories that count and calories that don't and is also the place where diet foods and drinks are manufactured that have been "purged of almost all their suddenly undesirable nutritive values." It's an entertaining travelogue—a nice place to visit, but you wouldn't want to try to lose weight there.

Regrettably, the land of real weight reduction is not a fairy tale country.

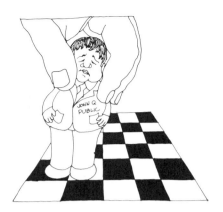

The Public Is the Pawn

Who falls for fantastic gimmicks, you ask? Who is letting himself be hoodwinked by meaningless promises? Who fails to read between the lines of those promising labels, written by advertisers who are adept at conveying what they can't actually *say* without encountering the long arm of the law?

Millions of ordinary Americans do—wealthy and poor, silly and sober, educated and ignorant. The "miracle" products keep on proliferating and sales are zooming. Farfetched testimonials and ludicrous promises don't seem to put off the buyers of today anymore than they did a hundred years ago. Let's take our own trip down through "Memory Lane" for a closer look at some of the advertisements that "sold" the public in their day.

The Not-So-Good Old Days

In 1885, The Wilcox Specific Company of Philadelphia addressed their advertisement to "Fat Folks," claiming that the use of their "Anti-Corpulene Pills" would cause a weight loss of 15 pounds a month. (Before you laugh, read the promises on the packages of today's diet aids.) The ad went on to assure the avid reader, "They cause no sickness, contain no poison, and never fail." Sealed particulars were available from the company for the price of a 4¢ stamp, but the advertisement was no more specific than quoted.

Another early remedy for obesity was called "Rengo," "Nature's Remedy." "The delicious juices found in Rengo are purely the products of nature herself." The manufacturer of this "cure" was Frank J. Kellogg, who produced an anti-lean as well as an anti-fat medicine. For his contribution to society, Mr. Kellogg reaped millions of dollars, which probably enabled him to support his four wives. The advertisements said only that Rengo "turned fat into muscle . . . perfectly safe and direct in its action," but this medicine is reputed (by later studies) to have actually contained thyroid gland substance.

During the "Roaring Twenties," many heavy-footed fatties were invited to waltz their weight away with reducing records. One can only speculate on the names of the tunes—and one imagines that the tempo was undoubtedly allegro! At least, that method involved some pleasant exercise and was one of the less extravagant suggestions.

Also in the early 1900's, The Corrective Eating Society of Maywood, New Jersey and New York, made such modest offers as "Eat to Live 100 Years" and "New Stomachs for Old." This could be made possible with "24 Boiled-Down Lessons" in a $3.00 book—*Eugene Christian's Course in Scientific Eating.* A later ad found Mr. Christian's course endorsed by Arthur True Buswell, M.D., who apparently had had a "recent talk" with Eugene Christian, "The eminent Food Scientist who has successfully treated over 23,000 people with foods alone!" This ad, under Dr. Buswell's byline, contained many exciting case histories, but no hints about the nature of the "Boiled-Down Lessons." For that, you had to buy the book!

This was about the same era in which the cereal manufacturers cracked down on constipation and other debilitating conditions which harmed the natural beauty of the human face and form. Post's Bran Flakes explained that, if you prized beauty, you had to obey "Nature's Law," because "Faulty Elimination is the greatest enemy that beauty knows." Pillsbury's Health Bran was "one of the family" and would correct the causes of "Brain Fatigue" which the advertisement's text revealed as due to constipation. The Borden Company published "Health Crusade Articles" to alert the American public to the threats and dangers of malnutrition. Postum explained why "Strong, vigorous, robust men" crack under pressure. "Borrowed Energy Must be Repaid . . . Try Postum for 30 days" et cetera.

In 1928, the Dietetic Research Department of the California Fruit Growers Exchange in Los Angeles spread the news about "Acidosis," the word they said was on everyone's tongue, (now that the problem of constipation had been solved, one assumes). The Fruit Growers Exchange was plugging something called the

"Orange-Lemon Paradox." Although acid, citrus fruits were claimed to be "correctives" of Acidosis, because "their effect in the body is *alkaline*." The ad listed "Acidosis Symptoms" so that you could check yourself. (Actually, this malady is an abnormally high concentration of acid in the blood and body tissue.) "Headache, sour stomach, biliousness, nausea, children's upset stomach, nervousness, sleeplessness, high blood pressure, acid perspiration, acid mouth, acetone urea, acid urine, and coma" were the symptoms. "Women and men desiring to reduce must be doubly careful to avoid Acidosis," the ad went on to say, "If you feel 'under par,' send at once for a free copy of our book, *Telling Fortunes with Foods*. If your case is in any way abnormal, consult your physician." (It's difficult to imagine a case involving coma which would not be considered abnormal.)

The obese of the early 1900's were also assured of instant fat disappearance and marvelous bodies through the use of vibrating belts (1928) and spot reducers (1913-1923), which guaranteed to make the fat melt away under the skin of whatever portion of the body to which you applied the machine, while giving you, in addition, "a perfectly healthy body." Electric Massage (1913) not only aided your health, gave instant relief to "headaches, neuralgia, rheumatism, backache, lumbago, scalp disease, falling hair, sore feet, tired feeling, nervousness, sleeplessness, paralysis, and other nervous ailments," but also, as a kind of added bonus, made your hair "luxuriant." The Home Electric Massage Battery enabled you to achieve all this through "the magic power" of the "radiance of faradic electricity." You were encouraged to take advantage of the "benefits of faradism at a price you can easily afford."

Perspectives—Yesterday, Today, and Tomorrow

To those of you who may think, "We've come a long way, Baby," and that people are more discerning now, we suggest that you take a cold, hard look at the current advertisements and blurbs for faddish and foolish diets, special diet foods, drugs and dietetic aids, effortless exercise and slenderizing machines, the suddenly-popular massage parlors and health spas. And, today, what is a home without a portable sauna bath? One wonders how *this* generation is going to appear to *its* grandchildren.

The wisest of men have, at some time or other, succumbed to a wild theory or two. In the First Century, A.D., Dioscorides, the Greek physician, believed that the liver of an ass would cure epilepsy and a potion made of grasshoppers would relieve disorders of the bladder. Pliny of Ancient Rome was convinced that the foot and snout of a hippopotamus would increase sexual potency. Way back in the Third millennium B.C., Egyptians fed garlic to the workmen busy on the Great Pyramids, in order to strengthen their bodies. (Garlic is pretty potent stuff and may indeed have made those huge blocks of stone easier to haul.)

Foods and herbs have long enjoyed medicinal (or poisonous) reputations. The French, thinking the tomato, which was cultivated in Central and South America and introduced to Europe by the Spaniards, to be an aphrodisiac welcomed it as the *pomme d'amour* (the love apple). The English and Germans, on the other hand, regarded it as poisonous as its deadly relative, nightshade. It wasn't until 1820, when Robert Gibbon Johnson stood on the steps of the Salem County Courthouse in New Jersey and, before a gaping audience, ate a whole tomato, that the tomato became an acceptable food in the United States.

Oysters, oranges, lemons, apples, peaches, pumpkins, carrots, cucumbers, and parsley (if transplanted) have all been considered, at one time or another, as dangerous foods for human consumption. At other times, certain foods were endowed with special powers. Cato the Elder found healing properties in the common cabbage.

The dangers of promoting one food generally reside in the exclusion of others, needed to make up a balanced diet. We have faddist diets today which come close to being dangerous because of their emphasis on one type of food, such as the Macrobiotic Diet.

In Early America, natural Indian medicines enjoyed popularity. The Indians did have a knowledge of native healing herbs and foods, but these bore little relation to the "Indian Cures" promoted by white men —one such was an "Indian Compound" made of "Honey, Boneset, and Squills" touted as a cure for "coughs, colds, and all affections of the throat and lungs." Boneset *(eupatorium perfoliatum)* was a commonly used remedy of the time. An infusion of this medicine would surely make the patient upchuck. We can only speculate on the medicinal properties of "Squills."

"Nature will castigate those who don't masticate," said Horace Fletcher. Seaman, art student, reporter, opera company manager, manufacturer of printers' inks, importer of Oriental silks and curios—Fletcher had pursued all of these careers, and such an active life had, he believed, left him pretty well worn out at the young age of 40. Although he was only 5 feet, 6 inches tall, Fletcher weighed 217 pounds. The least exercise speeded up his heartbeat and shortened his breath.

Ever the do-it-yourselfer, Horace Fletcher took up the study of nutrition in the early years of this century. In the course of his reading, he came across the tidbit that Prime Minister Gladstone had once remarked that because man has 32 teeth he is meant to chew every mouthful of food 32 times. Captivated, Fletcher coined his catchy "castigate-masticate" phrase. Of course, chewing is healthful. It stimulates the digestive juices and is very much to be recommended to anyone trying to lose weight. Most overweight people eat too fast. Fletcher, however, went a little overboard with this. He chewed so hard—and ate so little—that he lost 65 pounds in short order.

Was he taken seriously by the public? "Fletcherism" and "Fletcherize" became national by-words as everyone picked up the rhythm of Horace's jaws. West Point Cadets, John D. Rockefeller, Jr., Thomas Alva Edison, scientists at several universities here and abroad, all chewed and endorsed "Fletcherism." After his death in 1919, however, the craze slowed and finally disappeared.

In our own time, we have a few theories that come under the heading of "folklore." Never mix milk with pickles (unless you're pregnant). In Boston, brown eggs are considered more nutritious than white.

And, not long ago, the ghost of Horace Fletcher returned. One health cult advocated chewing every mouthful of food at least 50 times, recommending as desirable 100 or 150 chews. A Japanese girl reportedly chewed an onion 1,300 times, which may have strengthened her jaws if not her digestion.

Not all "wild ideas" turn out to be incorrect, but most of them do. We have a few ideas about dieting around today that have withstood the test of time admirably. And we have lots of others that ought to be viewed as objectively as possible—how will they look to readers 50 or 100 years from now?

In June of 1973, *Time Magazine* felt compelled to present the sophisticated American readership with an essay entitled "The Uncommonness of Common Sense." ". . . by mid-century" says the author, Stefan Kanfer, "sense was no longer common. Today the American public can be intimidated by those who ask Chico Marx's question: 'Who you gonna believe, me or your own eyes?'" Of the diet scene, Kanfer writes, "Only the commonsensical, apparently, have concluded that the less they eat, the lighter they weigh. Or that the more they exercise, the more fit they feel." But what he really sees is that "overweight Americans still seek an easy way to play the scales."

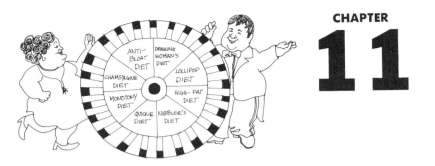

Fat Chance

The fact that craze diets are reaching epidemic proportions is clearly exemplified by the amount of space given to them by national magazines in recent years. Space means money, in magazine circles, and five or six pages (or more) in every issue represent a considerable financial investment.

"Between March 1969 and February 1970," writes Robert Sherrill in *Today's Health* (August, 1971), "26 diet articles appeared in *Harper's Bazaar, Mademoiselle, Good Housekeeping, Ladies' Home Journal, Vogue, Seventeen, and Redbook*." During the next year, these same magazines, says Mr. Sherrill, featured 38 more diet articles, "including sage and relevant advice on 'Dieting by Computer,' 'Chewing Your Way to Health, Sexual Vitality, Peace' (Fletcher again?),

'Hot Dog Diet the Three Star Way,' and, under a joint by-line, 'We lost 409 Pounds.' " It is ironic that today many of these same magazines helpfully devote many pages to warnings about the dangers of these same diets.

Regrettably, they are late with their warnings. The anxious, rotund reader is still following the fad rather than heeding the caution. If he can't find a crash diet in his favorite magazine, he can most certainly find several in the books on the shelves of his local bookstore. Let's take a closer look at some of the fabulous diets that have swept the country by storm.

Back in October of 1961, *McCall's* published "How to Lose Seven Pounds This Week," by Ruth West. The diet was described as "unorthodox" but "effective and sound," "a countdown diet," and "a double-barreled diet." "Countdown," because it was compared to diets "the astronauts go on . . . based on the theory of low residue, calculated to get you ready for a great occasion *fast.*" (The "great occasion" turns out to be "Christmas holidays, or an important party, or a tropic-vacation-cum-bathing-suit" affair. Vanity is still one of the most effective incentives the media can offer.) The diet was called "double-barreled" because, along with counting calories, you also counted sodium content. The basic ingredient of the diet was egg noodles, buttressed by fruit and juice, cheese, sliced almonds or cinnamon crunch, coffee or tea (without cream or sugar). The calorie count averaged 206 to 310 per meal with the portions allowed. In addition, Miss West promises, "You *can* eat these foods three times a day." (emphasis ours)

Giving up salt was the best thing about this diet.

Enough sodium exists in the foods of a well-balanced diet so that no extra sprinkling should be necessary. But this was hardly a well-balanced diet by any stretch of the laws of nutrition. Maybe you gave up sugar in coffee and tea, but you *were* having that sugared cinnamon crunch! And the main staple of the diet was a carbohydrate food—the most difficult kind of food on which to lose weight. Vegetables were excluded, meaning that your body was denied an important source of the total nutrition it needs. Less than 1,000 calories a day, it was a semi-starvation diet, as any carbohydrate diet would have to be. Anyway, the monotony of the fare would probably have turned your appetite off while you busied yourself with getting ready for that "great occasion."

If you only wanted to lose five pounds in six days, you could have turned to the January, 1960 issue of *Coronet* and drawn on the talents of Princess Alexandra Kropotkin. "Her highness" recommended that her readers become rice eaters, because in her world travels, she had "always been impressed by the slender form and active grace of the average Oriental—Hindu, Japanese, Chinese, Malayan—all of whom are rice eaters." Since she did meet "some overplump Orientals—including the rajah of what used to be a fabulous principality in India," it comes to mind that the slender Oriental might have enjoyed becoming "overplump," too, if he could have afforded it.

Not to negate the value of rice per se, the Princess presented no evidence for the value of rice in *reducing,* although she did emphasize its "cosmopolitan flavor." Alluding to a pamphlet written by Dr. Walter Kempner of Duke University called *Friendship on the Rice*

Diet, Princess Kropotkin remarks, "I am certain that stomachs overladen with heavier starches and with fats must be vulnerable to bad temper as well as lethargy. I've observed that all over the world." On the strength of this penetrating testimonial, one might recommend that world leaders and U.N. representatives immediately take up a rice diet, but, for those who wish to reduce, something a little more well-rounded is in order.

Apparently, when diet crusaders get turned on to one food at the expense of others, that food appears at every meal. The design may be to get you "fed up" rather than "fed." However, the idea should not be to barely skim by on 1,000 calories of starch foods, which should peel off a few pounds. What you should aim for is to turn from what you've been eating to a diet that will keep nourishing your body while it sheds unwanted fat. When you've reached your goal weight, you simply readjust portions to maintain that weight rather than reverting to your earlier habits. It's not enough to get by with that "satisfied feeling" from eating starches, while your body is starved for vitamins, minerals, and protein.

The really confusing thing for Coronet readers, though, is that, only a year earlier, they had been presented with Dr. Richard Mackarness' "Feed Yourself Thin" diet, in which rice which Princess Kropotkin enthusiastically recommended for every meal, was strictly a taboo food!

In *The Teen-Age Diet Book,* 1958, Ruth West tells the young people how they can lose three pounds in three days with the "Jet-Start Diet." For three days, three times a day, they could have eight ounces of tomato juice, three hard-cooked eggs, four rye or wheat wafers, black coffee or tea. That's about 313 calories a meal. Since both diets proposed by Miss West (also the author of the egg-noodle wonder) are supposed to strip off about a pound a day, at least the arithmetic is consistent. But let's do a little math of our own.

First of all, the caffeine, while it provides zero calories, will elevate the insulin level and make you hungrier than you'd be without it. Secondly, in three days, on this nicely-balanced diet, you would have consumed 72 ounces of tomato juice, 27 eggs, and 36 wafers. If nausea didn't set in, it would be a miracle.

On the bright side, active teenagers were allowed a 20-calorie serving of a green vegetable once a day, and they could chew celery or the nutritious eggshells, if they wished!

In 1965, there was another batch of fabulous diets. London gave us the "Eleven and a Half Cents Per Day" diet, which, as Peg Bracken points out, would be 38 cents in the United States. The British were encouraged to dine royally on this diet which "meets all nutritional needs:" a scant pound of self-raising flour (eight cents), two ounces of lard (two cents), quarter-inch carrot (one cent), and one and a half cabbage leaves (half a cent). You were directed to make a kind of stew with the carrot, cabbage, and some water (no cents?) and mix the flour and lard into dumplings. Then try to slide the whole mess past your taste buds.

That same year gave us Dr. Broda O. Barnes' "Bacon and Eggnog Diet"—although fatty, it was guaranteed to make you skinny. Dr. Barnes declared, "No heart attacks have occurred during the past 25 years among my patients on a diet high in saturated fats," and added, "food faddists" and conservative health experts who had been advocating polyunsaturated fats and the consumption of less high-fat meats to minimize the chances of heart disease were wrong. Dr. Barnes pointed out that Eskimos and one tribe in Northern Africa exist on a saturated fat diet and don't have heart attacks.

The diet consisted of: Breakfast—bacon, eggs, and a peeled orange (for vitamins), plus sugarless coffee or tea. Lunch—Eggnog made from one pint of whipping cream, one egg, vanilla, nutmeg, and non-caloric sweetner. Dinner—the same as lunch. *Bon appetit!*

The "Mayo Egg Diet," which apparently sprang from somewhere other than the Mayo Clinic, since that institution disavows it adamantly, claims to achieve weight loss through some magical changes in body chemistry due to the large number of eggs the diet includes. (You're probably beginning to see why the Mayo Clinic disclaimed this one.) You can eat all the eggs and bacon you desire, but you must have grapefruit at least three times a day. That's part of the magic, too.

The interesting thing is that you *can* lose weight on any of these diets. You will probably get so bored with the lack of variety that you will not overindulge in any food the diet permits. But the minute you go off this kind of specialty diet and begin to eat normally, you will begin to gain back the weight you have lost. Your taste buds will be starved for the "forbidden foods," and your body will be starved for nutrition.

For the truly desperate, Steven M. Spencer offered

a number of "desperate measures" recommended by obesity experts, in an article which appeared in a 1968 *Saturday Evening Post.* Dr. Garfield Duncan, University of Pennsylvania, proposed total fasting for two weeks when "everything else has failed." Dr. Duncan admitted that there could be complications on this regimen, that it should be administered in a hospital, and shouldn't extend much over two weeks. His caution was probably inspired by the fact that there have been a few deaths during extended periods of starvation even in hospitals.

A second desperate measure described by Spencer is Dr. Walter Kempner's "rice diet" at Duke University Medical Center, a four-month program whose medical fees and laboratory work came to around 150 dollars per week six years ago. That was a high price for rice! This diet probably works because, for all those months, you don't have time or permission to go to your local deli for a snack. You take all your meals at a "rice hut," and, if you've been very, very good, they add a few goodies to the rice.

The most desperate of all measures for the "hopeless" that Mr. Spencer's article describes is the surgical by-pass, in which 18 feet of intestine are cut out to reduce "nutritional absorption," attended not only by physiological risks and discomforts, such as several months of persistent and excessive diarrhea, but, in essence, the patient has "signed a contract" to short-change his body of nutrition for the rest of his life.

These measures are not only desperate, and probably foolish, but very expensive, in more ways than one. Since obesity may be a symptom of psychological disturbance as well as a physiological aberration, one cannot help but wonder how else the physical body will manifest its dissatisfactions at having only the physiological aspects of the total problem treated—and at an incredibly fast pace!

Slower, less amazing methods give the mind a chance to adjust to the "new person" who will emerge from the old when a great deal of weight is lost. Such methods may not get written up in a magazine, but they certainly would be safer and more comfortable.

It appears, however, that Americans will try diets and procedures like the ones described no matter how boring or dangerous they turn out to be. The admonition included in many published diets that the individual consult his physician and have a medical examination before starting the "recommended" diet regimen is *pro forma,* put in for the protection of author and publisher. They know most people won't bother to get a physical check-up and will just plunge right into these programs. Meanwhile, the inventors of these new diets achieve fame and wealth, and eventually appear on the "Today Show."

"Make Mine Vanilla"

For those who are not really feeling desperate but just want to trim away a few extra inches, without embarking on a costly medical program or counting and measuring lettuce leaves and cottage cheese, manufacturers developed the liquid formula diet. In 1960, 20 million Americans reduced their pocketbooks by more than 100 million dollars (some estimates reach as high as 750 million dollars) on formula diets of the Metrecal variety. After Metrecal came out in 1959, over 100 national and local brands of similar products appeared on the market.

There are several ways to use the formula diet. You can take it to replace one meal a day—lunch, perhaps. You can drink the formula for two meals a day. Or you can replace all your meals with four meals of formula, in which case you will be getting a pre-measured, "nutritional," perfectly-even 900 calories per day, without any of the fuss and bother of broiling chicken and chopping up salad. (Spartans can exist on three meals of formula, a total of 675 calories per day.) It's easy to carry no matter what your employment, and there are no dishes to clean up afterward. It's ideal for a picnic, because even the ants won't touch it. Nothing more convenient has been developed since Nature presented us with mother's milk.

One of the problems with this diet is that it is dreadfully boring—and the monotony of it, even if you add a stalk of celery for flair, makes it unsuitable for long-term use. If you are taking a liquid formula to replace all your meals each day, you may have elimination problems, because, after all, your system was designed to use solid as well as liquid foods.

It's not that the manufacturers haven't tried to deal with the ennui of it all. First they provided the reducer with yummy new flavors of the formula (premixed or mix-your-own) like imitation French vanilla, imitation wild strawberry, and Dutch chocolate.

Then came new *forms* of the formula. For those who longed for solid food, Metrecal introduced cookies, in assorted imitation flavors. And for those who remembered hot meals with nostalgia, "dinners" were manufactured. Essentially, the ingredients and the calorie count remained the same.

Here is a list of the ingredients, fresh off a box of Metrecal lemon crisp imitation flavor cookies: Wheat flour, sugar, milk protein concentrate, 8.4 percent vegetable fat consisting of a blend of hydrogenated soybean oil and hydrogenated palm oil, corn syrup solids, dried torula yeast, invert sugar, ammonium bicarbonate, iodized salt, lecithin, glycerin, artificial flavor, vitamin A palmitate, calciferol, ascorbic acid, thiamin mono-nitrate, riboflavin, niacinamid, tribasic calcium phosphate, ferrous sulfate, D-alpha-tocopheryl acid succinate, pyridoxine hydrochloride, cyanocobalamin, calcium pantothenate, potassium carbonate, dibasic potassium phosphate, cupric carbonate, magnesium carbonate, and manganese sulfate. Just like Mother used to make! (Of course, Mother would probably have used a real lemon, but you know how fussy mothers are!)

The formula diet method does not concern itself with emotional factors involved in obesity and makes no provision for keeping the weight under control on a long-time basis. Not many people can deny themselves the appealing variety of foods for more than a few weeks. If part of the problem is that they like to *eat* (and most fat *and thin* persons do like to eat), formula meals are not going to satisfy dieters over the long haul. Even babies outgrow formula mixes in short order!

"Why Do You Go On Straining Your Willpower?"

Why, indeed?! "No longer will you be the prisoner of a dreadful, uncontrollable appetite and lackadaisical willpower," says this full-page ad for the 1-2-3 Reducing Plan. "Part of what we call 'magic' is a tablet you take a half hour or so before your regular meals. It combines a pure vegetable extract that has no calories and starts acting to give you the feeling of a contented, full stomach . . . EAT THE FOODS YOU LIKE like Veal Scallopini . . ."

Or, if you're not in the mood for Veal Scallopini, how about some candy? "THESE WOMEN LOST 509 POUNDS AND FOUND WORK, LOVE, SUCCESS, BEAUTY, EXCITEMENT, AND EVEN JEALOUSY. These women ate piece after piece of candy. Ayds Reducing Plan Candy, containing vitamins and minerals, no drugs. Taken before meals, Ayds curbs your appetite . . . Isn't it beautiful the way the Ayds plan works? Available in four delicious flavors . . . At all drug counters."

These are typical ads for what are called "reducing aids," which we've mentioned before. Take a real look at the back pages of your favorite magazines and the shelves in your drugstore and read the glowing "come on," text.

Since the fraud conspiracy case against "Regimen," most manufacturers include "diet instructions" with the products, so that they can't be accused of claiming that the products themselves cause the weight loss. Of course, the diets suggested are so low in calories that weight loss is assured with or without the "aids."

Currently we find such inspiring names as "d-minish," "Bio-Slim," "Dex-a-Diet," "Monodex," "Figure Aid," "Appedrine," "Slim-Mint," "Natural Proteins," and "Ayds Vitamin and Mineral Candy" in most drug stores. Many recommend a physician's okay before the consumer embarks on these quickie methods and some even list a few of the physical conditions which require extreme caution or preclude the use of these products. They are not harmful, if the directions are followed, but on the other hand they are not much help in shoring up a sagging willpower either. Remember, the law does not permit the sale of non-prescription drugs strong enough to be effective.

How To Be the Toast of the "Talk Shows"

"Give to all men the things they secretly desire, and you will succeed more than they will" could have been written about the fabulous diets which feature all you want to eat (or drink) of foods that used to be "forbidden" to fatties. "All you want" is apparently a magic phrase which, when it appears on a book jacket, destines the writer for fame and fortune. And that may be the reason why we see the phrase so often.

All the martinis you want, all the whipped cream, all the mayonnaise and cheese, all the steak and lobster, and all the bologna you can imagine. Nevertheless, a lead-in like this *will* get the author on television, either when the book sells a million copies or when the author is investigated for fraud.

But, whether he is called to the cameras to explain a dazzling new diet concept or hauled into court to refute charges brought to issue, public appearances tend to increase sales. "I don't care what you say about me," old-time politicians used to say, "as long as you spell the name right." The idea is so foolproof that now well known television personalities are writing diet books, possibly to "up" their ratings. Ed McMahon has a very amusing book out about his battle with the potato, and a popular comedian has recently published a book about the diet of raw foods that he and his family have been following.

There are diets in print which feature every "favorite" food which one can imagine, diets for every physical, emotional, and spiritual "taste," diets for all ages and places of national origin—there is no lack of equal opportunity in "Dietland."

In case you may have missed any of the more dramatic diets available to you, we offer the following list for your consideration:

Diets A to Z

A.

Air Force Diet (we haven't determined yet *whose* Air Force)
Anti-Bloat Diet
Apple Diet (*not* guaranteed to keep the doctor away)

B.

Baked Potato Diet
Bananas-and-Milk Diet
Boston Policemen's Diet
Bio-Feedback Diet Plan

C.

Calories-Don't-Count Diet
Calories-Do-Count Diet
Champagne Diet
Cottage-Cheese-and-Pears Diet
Communist Manifesto Diet (party food for the working classes)

D.

Diet-with-a-Friend
Diversion Diet (that's any crash diet containing different foods from the last crash diet you were on)
Doctor's Own Diet
Doctor's Quick Inches-Off Diet
Doctors' Quick Weight-Loss Diet
Drinking Man's Diet
Drinking Woman's Diet

E.

Eat-All-You-Want Diet
Eat-Fat-and-Grow-Slim Diet
Eat-More-Weigh-Less Diet
Edgar Cayce Diet (you're reincarnated skinny?)
Eggs-and-Cheese Diet
Eggs-and-Grapefruit Diet
Eggs-and-Tomatoes Diet
Eggs-Eggs-and-Anything Diet

F.

Feed-Yourself-Thin Diet
Fish Diet

G.

Grape Diet
Grapefruit Diet
Grapefruit-and-Eggs Diet

H.

High-Carbohydrate Diet
High-Fat Diet
Hypno-Diet (you will get thin . . . you will get thin . . .)

I.

Ice-Cream-and-Pound-Cake Diet (okay for lunch, terrible for dinner)
Ice-Cube Diet (snack on a bowl of nice, fresh ice cubes while watching TV)

J.

Jesse James Diet (permits robbing the refrigerator at midnight)
John or Jane Doe Diet (you don't admit that you're on a diet, which spares you from getting a lot of well-intentioned advice)
Juices Only Diet

K.

"Kelly's Blues" Diet (no potatoes)
Kitchen Resistance Diet

L.

Lettuce-and-Tomato-Semi-Starvation Diet
Liquid Formula Diets
Lollipop Diet
Low-Carbohydrate Diet

Low-Fat Diet

Low-Protein Diet, Combination (Low-Carbohydrate and Low-Fat)

M.

Mao Tse-tung Diet (a steady diet of rice and poetry)

Martinis-and-Whipped-Cream Diet

Mashed-Potatoes-and-Other-Sensuous-Foods Diet (feed your senses, fool your body)

Mayo Clinic Diet

Melon-and-Berry Diet

Monotony Diet (bores you to thinness)

N.

Nibbler's Diet

Nibbles-and-Snacks Diet

North Pole Slenderizing Diet (disclaimed by the Eskimos)

O.

Ocean Voyage Diet (what you can't keep down won't make you fat)

"Oh, Say Can You See . . ." Diet (features hardly visible servings)

Oils-and-Fats Diet

P.

Pass-the-Pills Diet (mostly stimulants and vitamins)

Poultry Only Diet

Pray-Your-Weight-Away Diet (for those who eat religiously)

Q.

Quickie Diet (all the food you can eat in two minutes, three times a day—improves your figure but not your table manners)

Quasi-Food Diet (leans heavily on synthetics)

R.

Raw Foods Diet (properly with zither accompaniment)

Revolutionary Diet (any revolution will do—just keep running)

Rice Diet (includes all the raw fish you can eat)

S.

Sardine-and-Lettuce Diet

Senior Citizens' Diet

Skip-One-Meal-a-Day Diet (or S.O.M.A.D.)

Swingers' Diet (you work it off right away)

T.

Teenagers Diet

Temptation Diet (actually works the same way as the Monotony Diet, since your selection is limited to one or two "tempting" foods)

Telephone-Call-from-an-Anonymous-Friend Diet

T.O.P.S. Diet (Take Off Pounds Sensibly)

U.

Unit Trading Diet (for higher math students only)

Upsmanship Diet (two versions [1] you try to eat less than the next person or [2] you try to eat more than the next person without being detected)

V.

Vegetables Only Diet
"Vilhjalmur Stefansson" Diet (lots of caribou steak and seal blubber)
Virility Diet (heavy on the wheat germ)

W.

Watercress Diet
Weight Watchers' Diet
Wine-and-Cheese Diet (in case your parents are Italian)
Workingman's Diet (behave for five days, go wild on weekends)

X.

X-Rated Diet (substitutes sexual activity for snacks)

Y.

Yogurt Only Diet (in case your parents are Bulgarian)
You're-Only-Young-Once Diet (eat now the things that will be prohibited to you in old age—a contrast with Senior Citizens' Diet)

Z.

Zen Macrobiotic Diet (all ten levels)
Zero-Calories Diet (or, no food at all)

As time goes by, we're sure you will be able to add many more new diets to this basic list. The main thing is that there *is* something for everyone, A through Z. We haven't included the Good Health or Common Sense Diet, because we're coming to that later. Meanwhile, let's see what's going on in the Zero-Calorie Department.

The Fast Way

An article in *The New England Journal of Medicine* for March 1965 reports that "An obese diabetic woman was subjected to intermittent therapeutic starvation. The fourth fasting period was terminated by idiopathic lactic acidosis and death. The unfavorable outcome of this case suggests that therapeutic starvation should be undertaken with caution." This 400-pound woman was the mother of seven children and she was in a hospital under expert surveillance during the time of her fasting.

It is surprising to learn the number of people who endure occasional periods of fasting—on their own—in order to "cleanse the body of toxins" and "start over." Possible kidney damage and loss of lean body mass is not taken into account, nor is pellegra-like mental and physical deterioration resulting from a vitamin B6 deficiency. They persist, with almost religious fanaticism, in their self-cleansing, inviting possible complications like hyperuricemia, orthostatic hypotension, and anemia, all of which have been the reported results of hospital fasts.

It cannot be disputed that the human body is often host to undesirable toxins, but is fasting an appropriate or safe remedy for unspecified "toxins" or for overweight? There have been stories of almost miraculous "cures" through fasting. In April of 1972, *The Miami Herald* reported the results of treatment by fasting in Russia. "Besides arthritis, advocates claim that controlled starvation will cure almost everything from eczema to hardening of the arteries. It is recommended for some cases of gallstones and pancreatitis. The method is used to treat schizophrenic patients and others with less serious neurotic afflictions—fears of crowds, darkness, strangers, infections and sharp objects, and it is effective for people who only think they are sick," this enthusiastic article declares. One imagines that many fears could fade into oblivion when starvation is endured.

"Hunger therapy" is not new. It was used in ancient Egypt, Greece, and India. From the 18th century, Russian doctors at Moscow University have been experimenting with the treatment. Of course, the patients lose weight, along with being cured of psoriasis and metabolism disorders and whatever else is being studied at that particular clinic, since the treatment lasts from 20 to 40 days. But once the treatment is discontinued, and the patient again tastes food, the weight is liable to go right back onto his body, since no new eating habits have been established.

Dr. Yuri Nikolayev, head of one of the clinics at the Moscow Research Institute of Psychiatry, warns that "the hunger treatment should be administered only under carefully controlled conditions. The patient and his relatives must approve the procedure, and the patient is thoroughly examined before the treatment starts." The Russian doctors do not seem to have considered using this treatment for obesity, and all reports center around disturbing and dangerous illnesses on which "fasting" has been tried as a remedy.

Some things are not meant for do-it-yourselfers. The human body is a sturdy yet delicate mechanism with many complicated processes still outside the ken of the layman. Extreme measures like long-term fasting are not even safe under hospital conditions, so they should never be tried on one's own, even if one can find a physician to prescribe it.

By learning to eat right and to eat the right foods, a dieter can bring his weight under control in a natural way without incurring problems that outweigh any dramatic change in his obesity. And, best of all, the results will surely be more long-lasting. T. Lawlor and D. G. Wells, writing in the *American Journal of Clinical Nutrition,* September 1969, report that "Refeeding was commenced gradually (after fasting). For several days the patients were fed a diet of fruit and milk drinks only, before they were introduced to a high-protein, low-carbohydrate diet. Despite this gradual introduction to eating, termination of the fast resulted in rapid gain in weight *in all cases.*" (Emphasis ours.) In their summary, they add, "in prolonged fasting (i.e., periods greater than 40 days) electrolyte disorders, protein deficiency, normochromic anemia and malabsorption of vitamin B12 were encountered."

The Slow Way

If you're a dedicated dieter, you've probably accumulated half-a-dozen calorie charts by now. Ironically, you probably bought the ones you have where most people buy them, in supermarkets right near the check-out register—and there you are with your cart filled with all the wrong "goodies!" The supermarket does want to sell you the booklet but doesn't want you to be deterred from buying those high-profit, high-calorie impulse foods.

In recent years, more sophisticated versions of the calorie book have been published, in paperback and in hardback, but the same problem exists whether you pay 25¢ or $12.50—if you own two books, you own two different sets of figures. If you have a bit of larceny in your soul, you'll "rob Peter to pay Paul" and search feverishly through every book until you find the lowest number of calories listed for one of your favorite snacks. If you do this in every case, you can wind up with a fairly low total for your day's intake, but what exactly will it represent in terms of reducing?

Most calorie charts are also rather vague about portions. A "medium serving" of chicken pie is four tablespoons to one person and half a pie to another. Some chicken pies have all chicken in them, and some have potatoes and other vegetables. This can get to be a very complex matter and the cause of many a family argument. One serving of corn chowder—is that a cup or a bowl? One medium peach—can you deduct 5 calories if it had a bruise on one side? One tablespoon of mayonnaise—was that level or full or heaping? Never has so much cheating been encouraged, except perhaps in the field of politics!

Probably the most amusing (if you have a grim sense of humor) aspect of the calorie charts are the ones that give you the count by the *pound*. It's very interesting to learn that a pound of French bread is 1,315 calories whereas a pound of Italian bread is only 1,250—but no one who is trying to reduce really thinks he can consume bread by the pound, anyway. At least, we hope not.

Ice cream, you scream, we all scream counting the calories in ice cream . . . Is a scoop of vanilla ice cream ¼ or ⅓ of a pint, or ½ cup, or what? When you scoop it, do you level off, or are you generous with yourself? If you were asked how many calories in a "portion" of ice cream, what would you reply? Let's consult our conveneint, indexed calorie-counter books!

No-Guess Calorie Counter, Bantam Minibook, 1969

(no brands or flavors given)

Plain	(fat content not given)	½ cup	145 calories
Regular	(10 percent fat)	⅙ quart	174 calories
Rich	(16 percent fat)	⅙ quart	200 calories

Food & Drink Calculator, Dell Purse Book 2666, 1967

Sealtest	(10.2 percent fat)	⅓ pint	176 calories
Sealtest	(12.1 percent fat)	⅓ pint	186 calories
French Prestige	(fat content not given)	⅓ pint	247 calories

The Calorie Counter for Weight Watchers, Pyramid Publications, 1969

(no brands or flavors given)

| All flavors | (fat content not given) | 1 scoop | 150 calories |

Food & Drink Counter, Dell Purse Book 2665, 1970

(no brands or flavors given)

Regular	(about 10 percent fat)	⅓ pint	168 calories
Regular	(about 12 percent fat)	⅓ pint	180 calories
Rich	(about 16 percent)	⅓ pint	200 calories

The Joy of Cooking, Bobbs-Merrill, 1953

(no brands or flavors given)

| Commercial, plain | (fat content not given) | ½ cup | 190 calories |

The Good Housekeeping Cook Book, Stamford House, 1949

(no brands or flavors given)

| Ice Cream | (fat content not given) | ½ cup | 200 calories |

A Documentary on Weight, Diet, and Exercise, Lt. Col. Robert
C. Drebellis, USAF, Rand Corp., 1966

| Ice Cream, vanilla | (fat content not given) | 4 oz. (¼ pint) | 150 calories |

Oh well, we didn't want any ice cream, anyway! How
about some nice fresh blueberries?

Of blueberries, one list says ½ cup is 50 calories,
another says 3½ ounces are 62 calories, another two
lists say 100 calories per cup. Still another list con-
fuses the issue with 43 calories for ½ cup, and our
favorite list reports that ¾ cup is only 50. But one
last list (we're sure it's a misprint) says ¼ cup is 85
calories!

Let's see now—with some basic arithmetic we
find three lists out of seven assign 50 calories to ½ cup
of the fresh fruit. With more sophisticated math, we
could equalize all portions, recompute the calories,
and come out with a fairly "accurate" average. Lucky
to have seven lists to consult, else we might have been
misled!

Dieters know that chicken, especially broiled or
boiled, is a good source of protein, if you have to
watch your weight. One book says ½ small broiled or
boiled chicken is 100 calories. But, just a minute—how
small is "small?" Checking another list, four ounces
broiled is 150 calories. Would that mean just the
weight of the meat, not including bones? Maybe a
third book will help! This one reports "flesh only,
broiled, three ounces, 115 calories." Then there's the
list with a specific entry "Chicken, broiler." Good,
that's what a dieter wants. But the breakdown is as
follows: "fried, raw, canned, boned"—these broilers

are neither broiled nor boiled! Don't give up, though. We have more lists. "Broiled meat only, four ounces, 155 calories." Next list, "½ medium broiler, 125 calories," and another, "Chicken, four ounces lean meat, 145 calories."

It looks as if the person with the most calorie books wins this game, if he chooses the largest portion for the smallest number of calories, and if he doesn't mind cheating himself.

The vague and contradictory calorie lists are very difficult to use as a guide to eating for weight control. As we have pointed out before, these calorie books rarely give information about the *kind* of calories which should be emphasized in a reducing program. So the calorie lists can only be utilized in a most general way, to compare foods as to their relative energy value (i.e., bananas have more food energy than tangerines). And a knowledge of calorie content must always be supplemented with knowledge of vitamin and mineral content as well as carbohydrate count in planning a diet menu.

The Revolutionary Way

There are revolutions, and there are revolutions!

Not long ago, dieters were inspired by the "revolutionary new Rockefeller Diet," reputed to have been developed by researchers at the Rockefeller Institute for Medical Research. If your obesity was simply the result of overeating, and not caused by glandular or any other physiological disorder, this theory was focused on working magic with the *balance* of the overeater's diet.

The revolutionary idea was to place the fat person, obviously a victim of his appetites, on a low-protein or "appetite-control" regimen. Why would this control appetite? Because, at the Rockefeller Institute, they had figured out that it is *the protein in one's diet which stimulates appetite*. (Keep this fact in mind when we get to the counter-revolution.) Supposedly, limiting protein intake to one small portion per day (and we *mean* small—one egg *or* one slice of cheese *or* one slice of chicken) would limit appetite correspondingly. This would eliminate "nagging hunger pangs" and provide "foods essential to good health and good eating."

No alcohol was permitted during the first month of dieting, but cream and butter were sanctioned. Breakfast, with three kinds of sweet bread, butter, and syrup or jam, sounded like a nutritionist's nightmare, even with the unlimited fruit juice allowance.

This raises the question of whether protein is really important in a healthful diet. Protein is made of carbon, hydrogen, oxygen, and nitrogen. Most of our bodies are composed of protein material: blood, tissue, organs, skin, hair, nails, bones, and body fluids. Even the brain and nerves are protein. Since body cells and tissue are constantly breaking down and wearing out, we need this vital food element for repair and replacement.

Protein deficiency can result in a number of serious diseases and disorders: anemia; lack of antibodies to fight off infections; lack of protection of the liver against poisonous chemicals; imbalance of water in body tissues; unhealthy swelling or dropsy; potentially fatal kidney disease; inhibition of the healing of surface sores, cuts, and bruises; breaking down of muscles faster than they can be repaired; unhealthy state of skin, hair, and nails; constipation; insufficient hormone and enzyme interaction with vitamins and minerals to insure proper utilization of nutrients for the body's needs.

The natural appetite of the body is only satisfied when sufficient protein is available in the diet. The appetite satisfied by a low-protein, high-carbohydrate diet would more aptly be termed "taste." This generation has been brought up with an acquired taste for starchy foods that has little to do with actual body needs.

Revolutions, as it happens, often incite counter-revolutions. Either that, or the word "revolutionary" itself has come to mean a vast amount of money in plus sales—sales to fat folks who want overnight results, because isn't that the way revolutions happen?

One of the hottest-selling books in the history of publishing is *Dr. Atkins' Diet Revolution*—it's right up there with *Gone with the Wind* and *The Bible!* Here's how it's advertised: "You can now command your body to melt away fat—and lose as much as you want." No pills, no counting calories, no strenuous exercises. You'll "feel better—perhaps better than ever before." The promotional material promises you'll "lose weight the first week and continue to lose until you reach the weight you want to be! You'll melt away inches from your measurements . . . right where you want to lose them! . . . This amazing book could help change your life! The week after you get it into your hands you could be eight pounds lighter and many times happier!"

What you have to do, according to this theory, is to activate your F.M.H., or Fat Mobilizing Hormone. Some medical authorities claim there isn't any such hormone, but Dr. Atkins maintains that there is, and it is a "genie" which will signal your body to start "living off its own fat."

Of course, you'll want to know how all this is achieved, and, here's the surprise: in this case, *it's carbohydrate intake which is causing your appetite to increase.* Once you're on a high-protein diet, you'll be able to eat until you feel stuffed . . . all the time . . . and still lose weight. Dr. Atkins starts his dieters on a "zero" carbohydrate diet, with a vitamin tablet to make up for the deficiences. Two small salads ("loosely packed") are all the vegetables or raw foods allowed per day. Fruit, of course, has far too many carbohydrate grams to be included in this diet.

We know many low-carbohydrate diets, recognizing that this element is an enemy to the obese, restrain the "gram count" to from 40 to 60 grams per day, enough to prevent unpleasant side effects. Dr. Atkins practically eliminates any carbohydrates, thus encouraging a state of "ketosis" in the body—(which is what other doctors have tried to avoid).

While everyone has been rushing out to his bookstore for a copy of Atkins' Diet, there have been some rumblings in the medical hills. Ronald Deutsch interprets Dr. Atkins' diet as not really different from Taller's *Calories Don't Count* and Stillman's *Quick-Weight Loss Diet.* The revolution, then, is not so new.

Dr. Taller's diet, while very low in carbohydrates (allowing gluten bread, three slices per day, and two helpings of vegetables with less than 5 percent carbohydrate content, but no fruits) did not eliminate them entirely. He suggested cutting down on salt and stepping up exercise. He also recommended that the daily fat allowance, if not taken in other ways, be consumed in the form of safflower oil capsules—because safflower oil is unsaturated and contains linoleic acid, which reduces levels of cholesterol in the blood.

Since capsules of safflower oil were often sold in close proximity to his book, he soon ran into trouble with the law. The F.D.A. declared this to be equivalent to the sale of an unlabeled drug, and seized the displays of capsules. (If only they had acted as swiftly with the dangerous diet drugs containing digitalis or amphetamines!)

Dr. Stillman's diet (his *chief diet*—because he has many!) contains no carbohydrates at all. It is suggested that you take a multi-vitamin tablet daily and drink eight glasses of water. He is also the author of the baked-potato-and-buttermilk diet, the juices-only diet, and other amazing "quick" methods. Definitely not hung up on balancing one's diet, Dr. Stillman declares, "INEFFECTIVE BALANCED DIETING IS USELESS" in bold type. It is his contention that quick and bizarre methods are the kind that appeal to the overweight, who will ultimately fail to lose weight on a sensible, balanced regimen. These authors both recommended a low-carbohydrate diet, and Dr. Atkins is, indeed, treading on very similar ground. His slight shift in emphasis—to getting a good case of ketosis going in the body—is the only really new theory he has to offer.

Ketosis, says Dr. Atkins, is a state about which

we all have a great deal to "unlearn." Low-carbohydrate diets which permit up to 60 grams of carbohydrate a day are deliberately warding off ketosis (the presence of large amounts of ketone bodies, chemicals which spill over into the blood and urine as a result of the incomplete metabolism of fats). This is a mistake, Dr. Atkins feels. As he puts it, ". . . for a carbohydrate-intolerant Mr. Fat to be in ketosis . . . is a signal for rejoicing. It is a sign that the unwanted fat is being burned up as fuel . . . Of course, if you are in ketosis after prolonged starvation or because you are a diabetic out of control, it has a different aspect. Then it indicates the presence of acidosis—and that is a danger signal . . . There is no acidosis when ketosis occurs as a normal concomitant of this diet."

And how has the medical world reacted to this confident statement? The American Medical Association's Council on Foods and Nutrition labeled his book "unscientific and potentially dangerous to health." Dr. Stare of Harvard is quoted as saying, "The Atkins diet is nonsense . . . Any book that recommends unlimited amounts of meat, butter and eggs, as this one does, is, in my opinion, dangerous. The author who makes the suggestion is guilty of malpractice." Dr. Jules Hirsch, a specialist in nutrition at Rockefeller University, calls the book "the most unutterable nonsense I ever saw in my life." Dr. Neil Solomon, who has his own diet book out (it didn't sell as well) declares that the Atkins diet develops bad eating habits in the American public." But, worst of all, the A.M.A.'s sixteen page report on Atkins found his diet "without scientific merit" because "there is no evidence advanced that controlled studies were ever carried out to validate the observation that weight can be lost by sedentary subjects who consume a carbohydrate-poor diet providing 5,000 calories a day."

Dr. Atkins, while fighting back on many points, is sorry about one thing: "I'm sorry about (recommending) the diet during pregnancy. I now understand that ketosis during pregnancy could result in fetal damage."

It is interesting to note that his collaborator in this book was Ruth West (remember the egg noodle diet? . . . this was a change of heart for Miss West!) who came away from the business deal with the largest percentage of the profits, although receiving little acknowledgement as co-author (just a note on the inside title page). Miss West can chuckle all the way to the bank as Dr. Atkins fights for his integrity on the late night T.V. shows.

Heaping coals on the fire, the Medical Society of the County of New York called the diet "not new, not revolutionary, not miraculous and grossly unbalanced." They also noted that the dangerous effects of an extremely low-carbohydrate diet include weakness, apathy, a tendency to faint, excess uric acid in the blood (a precursor to gout), excess blood fats (a precursor to heart disease), loss of calcium, and, in persons with kidney disease it can cause kidney failure.

As if that weren't enough trouble, Dr. Atkins was implicated with the Cumberland Packing Corporation in the sale of cyclamates after they were removed from the market in 1970. Both names appeared on the packages which could be purchased without a prescription at the Cumberland address. Dr. Atkins feels the case against cyclamates is unfair, and "stuck his neck out" for the sugar substitute because he is an "idealist," he explains.

It is perfectly true that Americans consume many more carbohydrate foods than they really need, but before cutting this element out of the diet altogether, it is important to examine the real role of carbohydrates in the daily diet. We know they function as an "energy source, to the brain and muscles, that the energy derived from carbohydrates is not nearly as efficient nor as long-lasting as that derived from protein, but carbohydrates are necessary. Cutting down below safe levels pushes the body to the limits of its tolerance. Any diet which is too far out of balance, which eliminates entirely any one of the three food groups in order to effect weight loss, is denying your system essential nutrients and short-changing your body's ability to function properly and to repair itself as needed.

So we're faced with the problem of finding just the right proportions of protein, fats, and carbohydrates for a healthful reducing diet. Since each individual is unique, one can't come up with exact measurements and apply them in all cases.

If you reduce your protein intake to about half the usual amount, you won't "save" much more than about 200 calories a day and your diet won't be as palatable. More importantly, you would be inviting the hazards of protein deficiency. Reducing fat intake (which is one thing the Weight Watchers' program does) would eliminate about 500 calories a day, but it could leave you feeling unsatisfied, and feelings of hunger would tempt a dieter to cheat. This is why so many diet experts are turning to the low-carbohydrate form of regimen.

Remember, too, that obese people often react with hyperinsulinism to these carbohydrate foods. People normally consume about 350 grams of carbohydrates a day, and this is much higher than it needs to be for optimum health. A sensible low-carbohydrate diet reduces the "gram count" to about 60. This could deduct 1,000 calories or more from food intake, without hurting the body's functioning.

Some of the diets we've explained (notably, the low-calorie diets) actually limit all three food groups, but experience has shown that obese patients can't seem to stick to this method long enough to take off very much weight. The long-term benefits, therefore, are questionable. Why can't they stick to it? Because it leaves them feeling hungry most of the time. The portions are too small, and the amount of carbohydrate in proportion to fats and protein is too high for the obese metabolism.

The most sensible approach seems to be to cut carbohydrates to a healthful low level, while taking a closer look at the *kind* of carbohydrates which are chosen for the diet. Sugar, which averages about 450 calories per day in the average diet and does nothing helpful for the body (in fact, does harm), could represent an immediate "saving." Since, on this diet, protein is going to be the most important food, one can cut down on starches, because extra protein will produce needed energy. The daily allowance of carbohydrates should be taken in fresh, raw fruits and vegetables, rather than in breads, macaroni, and cereal products, which have been so devitalized of wheat germ as to make them almost useless in the diet, anyway. Instead, use wheat germ liberally to balance out the diet. Sprinkle it on salads, whip it into egg dishes, use it to replace bread crumbs in meat loaf—that kind of thing! It has a very pleasant, nutty flavor. Of course, you can't expect to eat all you want of any one food while you're on a diet! It just doesn't make sense.

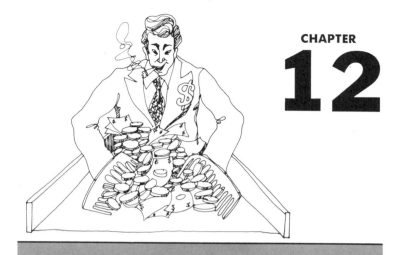

The Diet Business— Rakes in the Chips

Once upon a time, skim milk was used for hog and livestock feed, since it was a by-product of the more profitable portions of the milk. In her book *Consumer Beware!* Beatrice Trum Hunter reports, "When the dairy industry noted that the American public became calorie-conscious and cholesterol-anxious, it responded to changing consumer tastes, and diverted skim milk to this market." When this little pig-food went to market, dieters were offered not only milk they could drink without getting fat, but also cottage and other cheeses, ice milk, and sherbet, all supposedly proper foods for a reducing regimen.

Regrettably, the milk was skimmed by running it through a clarifier and cream separator before pasteurization to remove most of the fat, and fat-soluble vitamins A, D, E, and K were also lost.

On the bright side for industry, however, separating the milk increases the total milk profit since they use the leftover cream to make whipping cream, coffee cream, butter, ice cream, cheese, and other products.

Even dedicated dieters did not exactly go wild over cottage cheese in its natural state, so the milk industry offered them creamed cottage cheese, which, besides being more palatable, is also a lot higher in calories. (Again, some calorie books make this distinction, and some do not.)

The sugar content of ice milk and sherbet is usually quite high, making these desserts of questionable value to the dieter.

Skim milk itself has different food values, depending on the brand. One currently popular brand, which repeatedly advertises that you won't be able to tell the difference between it and the real thing, has evidently convinced Weight Watchers that there isn't enough difference. They have barred this brand from their list of acceptable diet foods.

Dietetic foods and synthetic sweeteners and seasonings are manufactured with the idea of motivating the buyer to purchase them rather than with a consideration of his total health and nutrition. Refined sugar, outside of giving you a brief "lift" for which you pay later in a more severe "down," has no nutritional value for the body, and dieters are wise to make this one of the first foods they cut from their food plan.

But some dieters miss the taste of sweetness so much they turn to artificial sweeteners and foods prepared with them. Saccharin is a coal-tar product, used plain as a substitute for sugar in coffee and tea, or in dietetic candy, soft drinks, and bakery products, where manufacturers find it cheap and easy to handle.

Researchers have shown evidence that saccharin can produce certain kinds of cancer in body tissue. The F.D.A., after reviewing the evidence in 1970 and admitting that there are still some unresolved questions, accepted the National Academy of Science's verdict that "on the basis of available information, the present and projected use of saccharin in the United States does not pose a hazard." By mid-September of 1970, however, the F.D.A. admitted that restrictions on the use of saccharin "were being considered."

Cyclamates (30 times sweeter than sugar) were an even greater boon to the food processing industry. This artificial sweetening, which does not lose its sweetness in cooking and canning, made it possible to increase the potential market for special dietary foods from chiefly diabetic use to include that huge mass of anxious reducers "out there" in the buying world. The history of cyclamates' role in food reads like a melodrama. We recommend Miss Hunter's book *Consumer Beware!* for a detailed report of how and why bans have been imposed on this questionable chemical product.

Chewing gum, which is about 60 percent sugar, is frequently recommended (sometimes by doctors) as an in-between meal snack for dieters. Again, the sugar is supposed to give your body a "lift" while the act of chewing satisfies your psychological hunger for the process of eating. Studies have shown, however, that chewing one stick of gum increases sugar in the saliva 3,500 percent while acting as a "pacifier."

Actually, the chewing and resulting salivation start the stomach muscles working and the gastric juices flowing. The stomach, expecting to receive food, is cheated and takes revenge by increasing hunger pangs. Chewing gum that has sugar in it is not good for your teeth or your diet. If it contains a substitute such as those we have already discussed, your body would be better off without even small amounts of these dangerous chemical substances.

Chewing gum is not an aid to digestion either, because, when healthy people chew gum, the acid normally required for digestion in the stomach is reduced for an hour's time.

As if this weren't enough, you may be interested to learn that a stick of chewing gum contains 25 to 30 ingredients in combination, some of which are "known allergens" and others of which are "suspected carcinogens." Once upon a time, gums were natural materials from tropical trees, but anything nature makes, man is sure he can improve upon (or at least produce at a greater profit). Besides the gum-base, sweetener, and the flavoring agent, you are also chewing coal tar colors, rubber, paraffin, plasticizers, resins, and a whole bunch of other tasty substances. Better double your caution while doubling your pleasure and fun with double-mint—the manufacturers are not even compelled to put the ingredients on the package, since gum is not considered a food. Yet, about ⅔ of a stick is actually swallowed when gum is chewed. That's why it gets smaller in your mouth.

Coffee and tea, without cream, milk, or sugar in them, are also frequently recommended as a way of filling the stomach between meals when you are dieting.

If you look these items up in your calorie counter, you will find an appealing "0" number beside them, which is how they came to enjoy this misleading reputation in the first place. Although they will pacify your stomach with a hot, non-caloric full feeling, that will last only a few minutes before even greater hunger sets in.

It's true that they don't contain calories, but coffee and tea do contain caffeine, which is an addictive drug. Aside from that, caffeine stimulates the production of adrenal hormones. This causes an increase in blood sugar, which is responsible for the temporary "lift" it engenders. Then, when the caffeine wears off, and the blood sugar plunges below normal again, which happens very quickly, the dieter will be even more tempted to fortify himself with a starchy snack.

When the coffee wagon comes around at ten in the morning, the best drink is a fruit juice like tomato, if you are very hungry. However, if you've had sufficient protein in your breakfast, you may just be able to work until lunch without experiencing hunger pangs. Another alternative is to have provided yourself with an apple or other whole fruit for the break.

If you must have coffee at this time in the morning, have a food or fruit juice with it for hunger, because the coffee is going to make things worse. It has no nutritional value, so it's only going to fool your body, for a very short time, into thinking it's consuming real food.

Caffeine is not very good for you anyway, and it's a better idea for the sake of a full-time, life-style, slim-down-and-stay-slim health regimen if the consumption of coffee and tea (plus cola beverages which also contain caffeine) be cut to a minimum, if not cut out altogether. If you feel you can't start the day without a cup, have the one cup but don't have two. Every little bit you avoid of the empty, nutritionless, and harmful foods will help with your dieting. All the healthy foods you begin to eat in proper amounts, like protein at breakfast, are going to help you to get slimmer while you remain energetic and good-natured.

Experimentally, caffeine has been demonstrated to cause genetic changes in bacteria, certain plants, fruit flies, and human cell structures, and the possibility exists that it may be a mutagen unfavorable to humans. Caffeine is also a poison. A drop of caffeine injected in the skin of an animal will produce death within a few minutes. An infinitely small amount injected into the brain will bring convulsions. The headaches and loss of efficiency a confirmed coffee-drinker suffers when he stops drinking coffee are typical symptoms of addiction—in other words, they are withdrawal symptoms. Coffee also raises the blood pressure, quickens the breathing rate, gives temporary physical stimulus, and so should be avoided by anyone with heart disease, angina, or high blood pressure. It is also detrimental to persons with stomach trouble, skin infections, arthritis, or liver trouble. Since caffeine is the chief irritant, a decaffeinated coffee can be used as a substitute, if needed.

In tea, along with caffeine, we have tannin acid amounting to about seven to 14 percent (depending on how far you stretched that tea bag). This acid, in concentration, has an unpleasant effect on the mucous membranes in the mouth and digestive tract, but, in the amounts found in medium-strength tea, it is not considered harmful. With the trend of communities to fluoridate water supplies, the tea-drinker should be aware that tea is extremely rich in fluorine. The combination of tea's natural fluorine plus that from a fluoridated water supply would result in a rather high intake of this substance. Tea, like coffee, will not alleviate hunger pangs but will increase their disturbing effect instead.

A dieter won't have to consume non-foods or chemical foods (such as the diet soft drinks) in order to get through the day, if he eats intelligently and concentrates on foods that are good for him. There are healthy and delicious foods and drinks that will provide him with the right nutrients for living a vigorous life while slimming down.

God Sends Meat and the Devil Sends Preservatives

Meat and fish of all kinds are some of the most vital foods to a dieter. They provide that all-important protein which he needs for energy, and, although according to a strict calorie count they are high, the body uses protein rapidly rather than tending to store it as fat the way it does with the carbohydrate foods. Protein "sticks to the ribs" and keeps the reducer from becoming too hungry between meals when the danger of eating starchy quick snacks is greatest. It has become obvious, however, that the food buyer has to be especially wary of preservatives and additives when buying meat and fish. Preservatives are designed principally to create the illusion of freshness through color and appearance and by retardation of spoilage. Additives can be preservatives and "extenders." These substances are used to insure the profitable sale of goods for the producers and vendors, not to benefit the consumer.

In ground meat, for example, it only takes a little carelessness for hamburger to become a host for rapidly multiplying bacteria. The color of the meat then becomes less than appetizing. What can the meat industry do? It can add coal tar colors, cochineal (a dye made from insect scales), sodium nitrate (which, in your stomach, is converted into nitrous acid), benzoate of soda (which the government warned us against in 1908), sodium sulfate, to mask the smell and give the red appearance of freshness.

This last additive has the characteristic of destroying the B vitamins and can cause a good deal of damage in your digestive system and other organs. Sodium nicotinate is another source of red color. Some localities have declared the use of this chemical as a food additive illegal, but 37 states say it's okay to use it.

Because ground meat is such an anonymous mixture, and so often used for diets, we especially want to point out that it is not an ideal food for dieters; other meats like chicken, fish, veal, or even slices of lean roast beef and steak are much to be preferred.

If you're going to use ground meat while dieting, have it ground for you by a butcher you trust, so that it will indeed be meat, not fat or a "horse of a different color."

Zen in the Art of Dieting

Many members of the younger generation have fallen under the spell of the Zen Macrobiotic Diet. The ritualistic trappings of this diet make it somewhat "magical." A Japanese import, the Macrobiotic Diet consists of eating patterns or "levels," ten of them. The partaker starts at the lowest level—cereals, vegetables, and animal products—and "purges" his way upward until he attains the highest level and subsists on nothing but cereals and limited liquids. Mystically, he has achieved a state of "well-being" when he can survive at the highest level.

Interestingly enough, the ideal is "balance" when working one's way toward the "top" of this unbalanced fare. Devotees seek to avoid being *sanpaku,* a sure tip-off that one is out of balance, revealed by the white of the eyes showing on three sides—on either side of the iris plus below the iris, too. This warning sign that there is a physical and spiritual imbalance is reported to have been exhibited by Marilyn Monroe, J. Edgar Hoover, Roy Cohn and others.

Followers of this diet suggest that balance and harmony can be restored by the Zen Macrobiotic Yin/ Yang "balanced" meal plan. New recruits will have much to learn. Something like a martini, the best proportion of foods is five parts of Yin to one part of Yang. Eggplant is Yin; strawberries are Yang. Every food is either one or the other, but before you begin to learn just where rutabagas, truffles, and *Fondue Bruxelloise* fit into this scheme of dieting, let's take a closer look at the nutritional aspects.

Macrobiotic dieters eschew chemical sugar and food that has been processed or treated with preservatives. This is very wise. They declare that natural unpolished brown rice is the most perfect food on earth, and it is indeed a very healthful food. Defenders of the system protest that their diet is misunderstood and misapplied. According to one of their spokesmen, they "try to eat in accordance with the laws of nature; cereal grains are the most abundantly provided by nature, so grain becomes the predominant food. Since rice is the largest of the grain crops, it is the basic grain for us."

Secondary foods are fresh root vegetables and legumes, and dried sea vegetables. In descending order, follow fruits, nuts, and fish or fowl. "Neither milk nor meat are recommended because 10 to 15 persons can be fed off the grazing land needed to sustain one cow." They insist that all the body's nutritive requirements can be met by this diet, even at the highest level.

Some groups stress this conservational approach to nature, whereby the emphasis is on what the land can produce, and other groups stress the medicinal and spiritual benefits of the diet's "balanced" Yin/Yang proportions: claiming cures for everything from hemorrhoids (on a number seven diet) to airsickness (by chewing on sesame seeds and sea salt powder—takes your mind off it, perhaps.)

The prime information center for macrobiotic diet practice in this country is probably Chico-San of Chico, California, an eleven-year-old corporation formed by former students of the "father" of macrobiotics in this country, the late Japanese philosopher George Ohsawa. Since its formation, through education programs, lecturing, and cooking classes, and developing a rice crop marketed at the rate of 3½ million pounds a year, the corporation has reached a gross sales of 2,500,000 dollars.

The number seven diet, which is cereals only and limited liquids, has been claimed to cure more than 80 ailments, including leprosy, leukemia, and cancer, in a few weeks and without benefit of medicine or surgery.

On the other hand, according to the A.M.A., enthusiastic adherence to the macrobiotic diet invites the dangers of scurvy and malnutrition. The restriction of fluids is, of course, a serious problem, as is the lack of fresh fruits and uncooked vegetables on most "levels" of the diet. On the tenth level, or the number seven diet, people can die, and some have. A 37-year-old woman died of scurvy after nine months on the diet, and a 24-year-old woman also died after several months on an "Oriental macrobiotic diet."

This is a diet with some good ideas in it, which, when carried too far, can be as dangerous as any we have reviewed, other than out-and-out fasting. No important food group can be entirely eliminated in a healthy reducing diet, although some will necessarily be limited. The intake of fluids must always be adequate to keep the body functioning properly—with the stress on plenty of good, fresh water, which, among other things, helps to combat afternoon fatigue.

"Don't Call Me, I'll Call You"

"A one to one relationship with someone who cares about your weight problem is important to those of us who are overweight," says Carol Teuscher, Director of Weight Control, in the promotional literature for this new telephone service for dieters. "A recent study undertaken by Weight Control, a Newton, Massachusetts group, has confirmed this through a group of dieters, many of whom were drop-outs from other diet groups. You are invited to participate . . ." You are also invited to pay a registration fee of 7 dollars and 50 cents as well as 2 dollars weekly to receive a daily phone call "of less than five minutes" from an anonymous diet advisor.

Who is this secret pal? Evidently, another of the registrants who is keeping a progress report on your problems and successes. And you, in turn, have the opportunity to call someone else once a day and advise them, even though, behind the "screen" of the telephone, you may weigh 400 pounds and have never dieted successfully in your life. None of you will know who the other is, in this game of "musical telephones" —only the Director will have this information.

Each of the registrants, who are kept busy making charts on one another, will only be known by his first name, but the very fact that you receive a phone call will give you the feeling that someone cares about you, although you may never actually meet this person. (With a plot like that, a soap opera writer could keep going for at least a year.)

When it's your turn *to be called,* the emphasis is on you and your problems. The "advisor" inquires about your morning weight and what you ate on the previous day. If you ate a lot, this could take up the whole five minutes, ". . . and then I had tomato *chartreuse* followed by a very small slice of *Gâteau au chocolat* which I just couldn't resist . . ." with only an occasional "tch! tch!" heard at the other end of the wire. But, if you've been "good" and there's time, other related problems can be discussed. When it's your turn to *call* an "advisee," the emphasis is on them and their struggle to get slim.

What kind of diet you choose and what your goal

weight will be is entirely up to you, but the organization does send you a diet to follow or will obtain one for you from your doctor, if you wish. If you decide to follow the diet Weight Control recommends, you can be assured that it will be "a diet based on your nutritional needs," even though you are not personally known to them.

They have sent you a questionnaire on the flap of the envelope which is already stamped and addressed for your convenience in mailing in the registration fee. There isn't much room on the flap of an envelope, so this is all they have space to ask: your name, age, address, telephone number, height, weight, and goal weight; your reason for losing weight (check one) health or beauty? and, lest we forget, "any medical problems?"

As a "bonus," Weight Control is currently offering, to those who achieve their goal weight, two weeks free attendance at a local Health Spa with a free massage thrown in for good measure.

Mrs. Carol Teuscher, a young housewife, conceived of the program "after eight years of trying to lose weight following my withdrawal from amphetamine and thyroid pills which I took on a doctor's prescription starting from the age of thirteen." For this reason, Mrs. Teuscher does not advocate nor encourage the use of diet "medicine," but those whose doctors provide special diets rather than pills for them are welcome to join the program.

Biofeedback Is Better Than No Feed at All

For reducers with a lot more than 2 dollars a week to spend, biofeedback and behavioral therapy may be the answer. Described in *Playboy* Magazine by Scot Morris as a "heart-stopping, eye-bulging, wave-making idea," biofeedback is a method of "tuning in" to your body's responses in a way that has never before been achieved, except by a few Swamis in India and, possibly, practitioners of Kung Fu. But they did it the hard way, without benefit of the biofeedback machine.

Basically, all the machine does is record your brain waves and read them back to you. You have three kinds of brain waves at work alternately: alpha, beta, and theta waves. Ordinarily, you have no idea which ones are in force at any given time. But, with the biofeedback machine, a soothing noise lets you know when you've reached the "alpha" stage, which happens when you are "daydreaming," that is, not conciously thinking of anything or trying to work out any particular problem or focus on one thought. On the other hand, you are not asleep either. You are just "drifting."

By practicing with the machine, you can learn to "turn on" the alpha waves at will (which is paradoxical, because, in order to turn on alpha, you have to be rather will-*less*). Being able to reach this stage whenever you wish has certain advantages, physically. For one thing, your blood pressure slows. And biofeedback has been used successfully with victims of high blood pressure who have learned to bring on the slowed-down alpha stage whenever necessary. Sufferers from migraine headaches have also been helped by learning to direct the flow of blood away from their dilating head blood vessels and into their hands while in the alpha state. It may sound crazy, but there is quite a bit of scientific evidence to support the success of biofeedback in treating headache. It is also used to control addictions, such as drugs and alcohol.

Biofeedback training is administered by behavioral psychologists, and some of them are willing to tackle any behavior problem, even overeating. This treatment will begin with a psychological profile and evaluation which may cost from 35 dollars to 70 dollars, and, if the profile indicates that you could be helped by biofeedback training, you will be scheduled for sessions with the machine along with an ongoing program of therapy with a counselor. Counselling is about 35 dollars per hour, and, the interesting thing is, you have no idea when you go in for this program just how many of those 35 dollar checks you are going to write.

If you can't pass the refrigerator without making yourself a ham sandwich, and you find yourself sleep-walking to the cookie jar nightly, and you are very, very rich, this might be an interesting program to investigate.

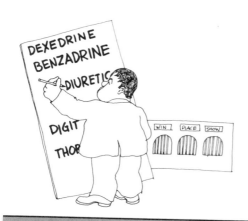

CHAPTER

13

Bet Your Life on a Rainbow Pill!

In a report to the Council on Drugs of the A.M.A., Dr. Walter Modell, Director of Clinical Pharmacology at Cornell University Medical College, said "Current pharmacotherapy for persons who overeat has limited use. Insofar as drugs are concerned, at the very best, their potential is secondary to the elimination of the cause of the hyperphagia (overeating)." In his concluding remarks, Dr. Modell added that drugs "which give assistance along the lines now available provide short-lived symptomatic relief only." They may be supportive to some degree, he feels, but the main emphasis should be on a carefully controlled diet and, if required, "some sort of psychotherapy."

Dr. Modell believes that obesity is "a consequence of a variety of non-related etiological factors" rather

161

than a symptom of "a specific disturbance in physiological function" or "a specific physical abnormality."

It is not at all unusual for results to be encouraging during the first phases of any reducing program. The difficulty is in sustaining the motivational interest in the dieter and in finding means to provide a substitute for the psychological satisfaction that food gives to the habitual overeater. Dr. Modell divides the drugs available for the control of overeating into seven helpful categories:

1) *Central Depression of Appetite*. This kind of appetite depression occurs automatically in the case of disease, as in hepatitis, or as an undesirable side effect of certain treatments, for example, a digitalis overdose. It causes weight loss, but, Dr. Modell points out, "even if it were safe as a therapeutic approach, it is not likely to be pursued because it is associated with distress."

This true central depression of appetite is accompanied by nausea or a sick sensation. Such an approach has no provision for prevention of regaining weight when administration of drug therapy ceases and the patient begins to feel better. "Such an effect of a drug on appetite," says Dr. Modell, "is not now consciously used in the treatment of obesity."

2) *Central-Stimulating Appetite Distractors*. Described as the mainstay of current pharmacotherapy of obesity, through the use of these stimulants, the patient's overwhelming desire for food is "distracted" by a sense of well-being or "lift." Amphetamines, unless given in large doses, "do not uniformly depress the appetite in all who overeat." While they have little or no ef-

fect on the patient's appetite, they may result in increased anxiety, increased physical and mental activity, and insomnia. They may dull the desire for the taste and smell of food (thus acting indirectly as an appetite depressant), and the increase in physical activity may also contribute a distraction from eating.

In themselves, amphetamines will not depress appetite to the point where patients lose weight unless they're also on a controlled diet. At best, the drug is a "crutch" which should be removed as soon as possible.

Manufacturers of the newer "amphetamine congeners" often imply that there's no connection between their compound and regular amphetamine, but their close chemical and pharmacological relationship can be easily demonstrated, says Dr. Modell. In addition to anxiety and insomnia, they also cause restlessness, excitement, depression, irritability, exhaustion, headache, dizziness, halitosis, dryness of the mouth, burning in the throat, nausea, heartburn, vomiting, and diarrhea.

There have been many cases of addiction to regular amphetamines reported. Since the body develops a tolerance for these drugs, their use can be effective only for a short period of time unless the dosage is increased. The newer drugs have not been in existence long enough for their addictive potential to be established.

3) *Metabolic Stimulants.* This group includes the thyroid drugs described earlier in this book. It also includes dinitrophenol (used briefly in the mid-nineteen-thirties) which increases the basal metabolic rate

without stimulating appetite and making the patient feel overly warm, as do the thyroid pills. Though weight loss occurred with dinitrophenol, the development of cataracts and other toxic effects led to it being abandoned.

4) *Sedatives and Tranquilizers.* Frequently, an emotional disturbance of some kind is the reason why a person overeats. If such a patient is sedated and tranquilized and the effect of the emotional disturbance is thereby diminished, he may feel less driven to indulge in food, according to Dr. Modell. Reports of effective treatment have appeared in medical literature, but the studies and data are as yet insufficient and inconclusive. In some cases, a combination of tranquilizers and amphetamines has been tried in the effort to combat some of the uncomfortable side-effects of the latter. The usefulness of this combination has not been proved.

5) *Bulk Producers.* Because the average overeater prefers to fill up with fats, proteins, and carbohydrates rather than bulky foods like cabbage, lettuce and celery, cellulose and similar materials have been suggested for use as a substitute for food. The theory is that, if the patient feels full, he won't eat as much of the fattening foods he has been consuming. Dr. Modell points out that this provides bulk for the intestine as well as the stomach, so it could never be taken in amounts sufficient for controlling appetite. Methylcellulose, therefore, has turned out to be neither an appealing nor useful way to control overeating.

6) *Purgatives and Diuretics.* The use of these drugs causes an immediate loss of water which is used to im-

press customers of health and diet courses with the effectiveness of the treatment. Since loss of water is not loss of fat and because the water will return to the body as soon as the diuretics are discontinued, these drugs are senseless and meaningless, except as a way of promoting profit for those who run courses in weight control.

7) *Miscellaneous Devices.* Dr. Modell comments: "What is strange, however, is that sweets (Ayds, R.D.X.) containing other nutritional elements in addition should have been introduced and should have their enthusiastic supporters... Weight loss through the use of such unscientific preparations can only be excellent proof of the importance of psychogenic elements involved and of the effectiveness of suggestive advertising."

Reducing aids, of course, rely heavily on the "Carbohydrate-jump," since some of them contain nearly all carbohydrate.

Dr. Modell's report was published in 1960, and we have quoted rather extensively from it to point out that this kind of information has been available for several years. One would assume from this that any drugs being given out today would be new, different, proven effective, and safe. They would not be the ineffective ones named in this report, as follows:

Amphetamines and Amphetamine Congeners: sympathomimetic amine-type, ephedrine, amphetamine (Benzadrine) sulfate, levo-amphetamine, levo-amphetamine alginate (Levonor), amphetamine resin complex (Biphetamine Resin), dextroamphetamine (Dexedrine), methamphetamine (Amphedroxyn, Desoxyephedrine,

Dosoxyn, Desyphed, Dexoval, Doxyfed, Drinalfa, Efroxine, Methamphetamine, Norodin, Semoxydrine, Syndrox) hydrochloride, phenylpropanolamine (Propadrine), phenmetrazine (Preludin), phenyl-*tert*-butylamine resin (Ionamin), and diethylpropion (Tenuate, Tepanil) hydrochloride. Phenylpropanolamine was also included in Regimentablets, Di-Dol, Rx121, and other "remedies" requiring no prescription. Another group—amine oxidase inhibitors and other so-called psychic energizers include pipradol (Meratran) and methylphenidate (Ritalin). Metabolic Stimulants: dinitrophenol, thyroid hormone, sodium liothyronine (Cytomel).

Sedatives and Tranquilizers: amobarbital (Amytal), chlorpromazine (Thorazine), rauwolfia (Raudixin, Rauserpa, Rauval), and meprobamate (Equanil, Meprospan, Meprotabs, Miltown).

Bulk Producers: methylcellulose

Purgatives and Diuretics includes various cathartics. Miscellaneous Devices includes Ayds and R.D.X. (Many of the reducing "aids" on your drugstore shelves fall into this same category.)

Some of these drugs are no longer used, a few have been outlawed for over-the-counter sales, many have always been available only by prescription, but the popular reducing "aids" are still with us (in some cases, under new names) because business is so good.

In the late nineteen-fifties, Americans were spending 1,000,000 dollars daily on reducing pills, capsules, tablets, crackers, candy, and other diet helpers. Most of the advertisements promised that their product would melt away ugly fat with ease. Meanwhile, a

Congressional committee was charging fraud against "questionable get-slim-quick product manufacturers which, according to the committee, swindled the American public out of 100,000,000 dollars a year. The Post Office was annually closing the mails to about 50 "fraudulent" reducing items. The F.D.A. was taking weight-less products off the shelves for technical "misbranding"—for claiming, for instance, that a product would cause a specific loss of fat in a definite amount of time.

In an article published in *Pageant* Magazine, Donald Cooley brought these facts to light and tried to divide the products into categories, commenting on their effectiveness, uselessness, or actual harm. He cited three main types: Before-meal-candies, lozenges, tablets, et cetera; stomach stuffers; and "preparations containing small amounts of active drugs." All of these kinds of "aids" are still available today, despite Mr. Cooley's best efforts to expose them. In some cases, the names have been changed to protect the guilty.

The first type are supposed to raise your blood sugar level so that you feel less hungry and will be satisfied with a low-calorie meal. The second type contain substances which, once swallowed, swell up in your stomach and, supposedly, make you feel "comfortably full." Your immediate reaction may be "yeck!", but these delicious non-foods are still around, and many people are using them. The third group includes drugs that are reputed to cut down your appetite in various ways: some claim to "flush the weight away," whatever that means. A careful comparison of the large-print "come on" and the small-print list of ingredients tips-off the wary as to just how exaggerated the big-type claims are.

The "before meals" variety are made of various combinations of skim milk powder, condensed whole milk, vegetable residues, sugar, flavoring, artificial sweeteners, and, in some, a few vitamins. What you're paying for is the manufacturer's thoughtfulness in providing this "magic" combination. The milk ingredients are the same as you find in powdered or bottled milk; the vegetable residues add little except bulk to the product; the saccharin, being a chemical sweetener, does not raise your blood sugar and has no food value. But, as Mr. Cooley points out, "Sugar does raise blood sugar levels quite rapidly." (Why not, one wonders, take a sugar cube and a vitamin tablet and save the money?) The sugars in these products often bear slightly camouflaged names such as "dextrose" or "sucrose." But it is actually the sugars that depress your appetite. That's why your mother always said, "Don't eat that candy now—it will spoil your dinner!"

Another magic ingredient is water or any hot liquid. The glass of water or cup of coffee that's recommended with a tablet or capsule will give you a slightly full sensation, temporarily.

The "stomach stuffers" contain vegetable gums and forms of cellulose that produce bulk. Labels describe the ingredients as flour, methylcellulose, carborymethylcellulose, and so on; the idea is to be impressive. Although these substances are supposed to fill your stomach with calorie-less bulk by swelling into a soft, jelly-like mass, much of the swelling occurs in the intestines instead, "beyond the reach of 'hunger pangs'."

In medicines, the main use of these substances is as laxatives.

The over-the-counter reducing "aids" containing various amounts or combinations of drugs are divided mainly into chemicals, diuretics, and anesthetics. The chemicals are intended to stimulate the nervous system. The caffeine in a cup of coffee will do as much (or as little) for weight control as the caffeine content of reducing pills.

Propadrine (phenylpropanolamine), useful for relief of hay fever or asthma, was touted as a "No-Diet Wonder Drug," an "amazing scientific discovery" that lets you "lose all the weight you want to without any kind of diet." Propadrine was not identified, however, except by the cryptic "PDQ-76." (Perhaps the initials stood for "Pretty Damn Quick.") This chemical is related to strong appetite-depressing drugs that doctors do prescribe in the treatment of obesity, but, in the amounts incorporated into over-the-counter remedies, it's too mild to have any real effect. If phenylpropanolamine is contained in reducing pills, the label must include the warning that persons with high blood pressure, heart disease, diabetes, or thyroid disease should use only as directed by a physician.

Ammonium chloride and other diuretics will rid your body of abnormal accumulations of liquid. Now you know why reducing remedies containing this chemical speak of "flushing." In the overweight person without an abnormal accumulation of water, the loss will be only of normal water, certainly not fat. A steam bath or a dose of Epsom salts might do the same thing.

Then there are the reducing pills that contain

benzocaine, "a local anesthetic useful in easing sore throats or sunburn. There is no evidence that it has any effect on appetite or food consumption," unless indirectly by stunning the taste buds so that nothing tastes good.

Dr. Joseph F. Fazekas published a paper in the *New England Journal of Medicine,* 1961, on anorexigenic agents (the word is related to anorexia and suggests the repressing of appetite). In his concluding remarks, the author commented, "It is likely that no such drug alone will ever cure obesity. The obese patients who have most satisfactorily responded to treatment may, in the majority of cases, be considered to be under temporary control, and are not actually cured, unless the psychophysiologic factors responsible for their excessive appetite disappear permanently."

Many of the drugs mentioned by Dr. Fazekas were also included in the Modell report. It would seem, therefore, that the use of such drugs should not have been continued, at least not until some laboratory evidence of their effectiveness was forthcoming. Despite the warnings of their more scientific colleagues, many doctors still prescribe these drugs in the treatment of obesity. The consequences have ranged from merely harmful to fatal.

Doctors do tend to prescribe drugs for obese patients during the early phases of treatment in hopes that the immediate results will motivate the dieter to continue his weight reducing regimen. As the Modell and Fazekas reports indicate, however, this has the effect of an only temporary victory, and, psychologically, for the patient, is not that different from the quick losses he can obtain from fad or foolish diets and health spas. These easy measures seem to increase the dieter's frustration and disappointment when the going gets rougher. He remembers the first pounds he lost fast and assumes he's failed again. In some cases, unpleasant side effects or drug dependency contribute more problems.

By the end of 1968, many injuries and more than 40 deaths had been linked to "diet pills." The thought comes to mind that there may have been many cases not detected and so not reported. Take abnormal births, for example. The *British Medical Journal* printed a letter in 1961 which reported on a patient who took Preludin during the first two months of pregnancy and gave birth to a child whose limbs were deformed. Two British doctors suggested that Preludin may have been a cause of other abnormal births.

In another case, an 18-year-old girl from Philadelphia, fighting to overcome an addiction to narcotics, told a reporter of the *Philadelphia Inquirer* that she became a slave to drugs through a weight control program administered by doctors and paid for by her mother. Introduced to reducing pills at the age of 12, she discovered, at the age of 14, that they helped to ward off boredom and depression. At 15, she turned to more powerful drugs and, finally, to heroin. This story appeared in print in 1966. One wonders how many other such stories never came to light.

It's difficult to understand why, with the reports appearing in research literature and the reports in the news media, doctors persist in utilizing drugs to reduce appetite, combining them with sedatives to offset the "high" from the stimulants.

In 1966, Rose Napoliello, having spent three

years in agony and having suffered many months with embolisms in the blood and heart and from brain damage, endured the amputation of both legs. The cause of the illness, the complications, and her subsequent death remained a mystery until it was discovered that Mrs. Napoliello, long a victim of rheumatic heart disease, had been taking a variety of prescribed diet drugs. The prescribing doctors agreed to an out-of-court settlement with Mr. Napoliello.

Darrell Holland, coroner of Effingham County, Illinois, said in January of 1968, "We have had approximately 14 suspected deaths from diet pill ingestion," and added that most of the victims had been young and died suddenly and unexpectedly. Dr. Samuel K. Lewis, coroner for DuPage County, Illinois, has said that he sees about one case every six weeks in which he suspects diet pills as the cause of death. Dr. Russell Henry, State Medical Examiner of Oregon, investigating links between diet pills and fatalities for several years, connected at least six deaths directly with reducing pills. One such case was that of 19-year-old Cheryl Oliver. She lost 40 pounds before suddenly keeling over dead at her desk in an Oregon State University dormitory.

In 1957, Representative John A. Blatnik (D.-Minn.) said, following a congressional investigation, that Americans spent more than 100,000,000 dollars during 1956 on weight-reducing preparations that had been found worthless and dangerous. Eleven years later, Dr. James Goddard, Commissioner of the F.D.A., testified that, until that time, the F.D.A. did not have sufficient evidence of a cause-and-effect relationship between diet pills and human suffering and deaths.

"Crashing" to Reality with Diet Drugs

Unlike the more harmful drugs, diuretics are merely useless in the treatment of obesity. Beyond rushing the nutrients through your system, cathartics will not send you to that Great Diet Workshop in the Sky. They may, however, impair the body's natural elimination processes.

Phenylpropanolamine was said to lessen appetite. It served as a psychological crutch without any actual effect on the desire for food. Ethyl aminobenzoate was designed to deaden the taste buds. Since the desire to eat is controlled by the appestat, an appetite center in the brain, rather than by taste buds, a powerful anesthetic which works in the mouth cannot lessen your yearning for good-tasting foods you remember.

Except for the very small percentage of obese persons who actually suffer from thyroid gland malfunction, taking thyroid extract to stimulate your metabolism will only step up your appetite, too, and give you a number of unpleasant or dangerous side effects. Since the early 1960's, researchers have been saying that the only indication for thyroid medication in weight control is hypothyroidism.

Another hormone administered to obese patients is HCG, human chorionic gonadotrophin, called a "sex hormone." Its primary advocate, Dr. A. T. W. Simeons, found in his experiments during the 1950's that it seemed to dissolve accumulations of fat and to reduce the size of the waist on patients he'd been treating for Froelich's disease, an illness characterized by sexual underdevelopment and extreme obesity. HCG is produced by the placenta during pregnancy. When his young patients ate normally, however, they lost no weight; it was simply redistributed. When he put some of his HCG patients on a rigid diet of 500 calories a day, they lost a pound a day without experiencing hunger pangs. Dr. Simeons now operates a clinic in Rome where he treats more than 1,000 patients a year with HCG anti-obesity therapy.

Word of Dr. Simeons' sex hormone treatment has spread, and it was estimated in 1968 that as many as 400 American doctors were administering this drug to their patients.

HCG is the same drug that has been used as part of the treatment that causes multiple births in previously infertile women. It seems inadvisable that anyone would take such a powerful drug merely to diet. If it must be accompanied by a 500-calorie diet to be effective, why not try the diet alone, or, better yet, a less rigorous diet?

Dr. William McGanity, writing in the *Journal of the American Medical Association,* warns that a 500-calorie diet is potentially more dangerous to the patient's health than continued obesity. Tampering with the hormone balance is also a hazardous affair.

In the March, 1964 issue of the *American Journal of Clinical Nutrition,* Captain Barry W. Frank of the Army Medical Corps reported that he had found failures resulting from Dr. Simeons' obesity treatment involving HCG. He also pointed out Dr. Simeons' own lack of support for his theory—no data regarding fat studies, fatty acid turnover, and the like. Dr. James H. Hutton of Chicago, defending Dr. Simeons, replied that a number of researchers had pretended to check the Simeons theory but had "modified" the procedure, changed the dose of medication, administered it at a different time, and the doctors did not see the patients. Hutton added that HCG enabled a patient to live on a small amount of food with little or no discomfort, enabled him also to take off weight where it should come off, and to experience "an unusual euphoria." Are these "benefits" truly desirable from a health standpoint?

The most dangerous of all the drugs used in diet pills is digitalis, a heart stimulant known to be fatal in large doses. While the number of doctors using HCG was estimated at 400 in 1968, the number of doctors using digitalis for weight control in that same year was estimated to be 5,000! Despite the general medical opinion that digitalis was useless against the overweight problem, some of the doctors who were using it were netting up to 2,000 dollars a day on their reducing regimens. This enormous profit may have made it more difficult for these diet doctors to comprehend reports about the ineffectiveness and dangers of using diet drugs. People continued to become ill and sometimes died as a result of treatment which included digitalis.

In February of 1968, F.D.A. Commissioner Goddard admitted before an investigating committee that F.D.A. had been aware of the risks in the thyroid-digitalis combination obesity therapy for more than 22 years, but took no action. Mrs. Dorothy Goodwin, attorney for the investigating committee testified that, to her knowledge, F.D.A. had not been concerned with the danger in diet drugs until recent national publicity brought them to public attention. (A month earlier, *Life* Magazine had run a feature story on diet pills, and public indignation was aroused.) Mrs. Goodwin stated, "When I first went to the F.D.A. in the latter part of

September (1967) . . . I was told that no one was working on the subject."

Early in January, 1968, the F.D.A. made some token seizures of thyroid and digitalis combinations, on the charge they were mislabeled, not that they were dangerous to health. F.D.A. confined its activity to two or three of the smaller producers. L. C. Tobin, president of one of the raided firms, Western Research Laboratories, angry at being singled out, said, "This was the basest, vilest, and most cynical form of headline hunting by a federal agency under pressure . . . We are one of more than 50 firms making some of the drugs, thyroid and a combination of thyroid and digitalis." He added, "These labels have been used for seven years and have been in the F.D.A. files for seven years."

The *Life* feature on diet pills mentioned earlier deserves a closer review. It alerted the public to the fact that there were an estimated 5,000 to 7,000 "fat doctors." About 1,000 of them were treating obesity exclusively, with five to ten million patients, selling more than two billion diet pills, and grossing a quarter to a half billion dollars a year.

Many of these doctors used a high-powered combination of pills that came to be known as "Rainbow Pills" because they were a variety of colors. While the drugs were not lethal in themselves when used in correct dosage for medical reasons, they were being "dispensed excessively and in dangerous combination" and they could, therefore, "become toxic, even fatal."

The "Rainbow Pill" group included most of the drugs we have been describing for their singular problems and side-effects administered *all at the same time:*

amphetamines, to suppress appetite; barbiturates, to combat the anxiety and sleeplessness caused by amphetamines; thyroid, to increase the rate at which the body burns up its food; diuretics, to dehydrate the body; laxatives; and digitalis, for which no logical reason has been given. *Life* finally explained to the public that "Certain diuretics, called thiazides, tend to cause great potassium loss, which in turn may make the heart so sensitive to digitalis that even a small dose can cause violent spasms—and death."

Life pointed out that there were "fat doctors" who do take precautions in treating their obese patients by giving them thorough examinations and prescribing drugs carefully. But they seemed to be in the minority and never became as wealthy as the fast operators. Reporter Susanna McBee visited ten of them. She admitted to being "a little on the hippy side, perhaps," but her picture, taken in a bathing suit one hour before her first investigatory visit belied her confession of even that much overweight. She was at the time 5'5" tall, weighed 123 to 125 pounds, and called herself "a reliable size 10."

In a six-week period, "traveling to nearly every section of the country," she went to ten doctors who specialized in weight problems. Although she had expected to be dismissed on the basis of having no real weight problem at all, "they welcomed me." One doctor congratulated her on "catching the problem early" (that must have meant, before it even developed); three of them did tell her that she didn't really have a weight problem, but *every one of them* gave her a fistful of diet pills, even though she never asked for them. "My 'haul'," Miss McBee exulted, "was 1,479 pills."

At no time did any of these doctors fully and frankly explain what medicines they were prescribing, and why and how they worked in the body, even in response to direct questioning from "patient" Miss Mc-Bee. Sometimes the name of *one* of the drugs was mentioned in a vague way.

Among the "fat doctors," there was no concensus on diet—some offered elaborate diets and some recommended eating anything a patient wanted. They did not agree on exercise or on liquor consumption. Physicals ranged from several tests to a mere weight and measurement check. "There was consensus, though," Miss McBee reported, "on one point: pills, pills, pills."

The Right To Ask Questions— and To Get Answers

As a patient, you have every right to ask what any drug is that a doctor prescribes for your benefit . . . and to demand an answer if evaded. It's your body which is being medicated. Answers to questions about the doctor's diagnosis of your condition should be answered forthrightly and honestly. The function of a doctor is to prevent illness or to heal it. Pill-pushing, theatrics, television appearances and writing diet books are all peripheral to this dedication.

The *Life* article also pointed out that many drug manufacturers were benefiting from the booming diet pill industry, but that the companies that made the most profit were about a dozen smaller outfits that distributed their products almost exclusively to "fat doctors." The Senate Anti-Trust Subcommittee subpoenaed the records of 10 such companies for the

1968 hearings. The drugs themselves, the article explained, "are produced very cheaply and some can be sold to doctors in wholesale lots at a cent apiece." Doctors charged up to 75 dollars a visit to treat obese patients, and some of them grossed nearly one million dollars annually.

Doctors who experiment on gullible patients and dispense diet pills haphazardly are only a few steps away from the "pusher" on the street corner. Either way, you can die of an overdose. Cases involving death from diet pills have been cited frequently in professional and popular literature. It should be clear by now that a reputable doctor will suggest a safe, gradual weight-losing program suited to your particular case, with full awareness of your physical condition and medical history. He will help you to work out a diet you can *live* with on a long term basis. If the doctor you go to tries to *con*vince you that you can do it easily and fast on pills, it's time to look for another doctor.

It is the thesis of Dr. Russell C. Henry, in an article published in *Nutrition Today* that, although some of these drugs seem harmless enough when taken alone, they have "a fatal interaction when taken together." Certainly none of the "fat doctors" whom Miss McBee investigated told her the exact drugs they were prescribing. How would a patient know if he were taking a dangerous combination or a harmless group, unless he asked questions and got answers?

The usual "rainbow" combination was a thiazide diuretic, a vegetable-type laxative, amphetamines or amphetamine-barbiturate combinations, thyroid extract, and digitalis. Sometimes a potassium supplement was given, and sometimes various combinations of hormones were used, including ovarian extract and anterior pituitary substances along with the previously mentioned thyroid. According to Dr. Henry, except for the thyroid-digitalis combinations, these drugs "have their places in the therapeutic management of diseases. However, by a combination of action and interaction, these rainbow pills are suspected of being responsible for the deaths of at least six women here in Oregon." The women, says Dr. Henry, were found dead in bed "after having been noted to have been enjoying 'usual' health previously. All were subsequently found to have been taking rainbow pills."

Positive proof is difficult to obtain on just how the drugs interacted in those who died. There are at least two known cases in which patients recovered and were cured of conditions (quadriplegia and respiratory paralysis in one case, and palpitations and other heart symptoms in the other) when they discontinued the use of the rainbow pills they had been taking. A routine hospital laboratory screening of the first patient had shown "a very depressed blood potassium level, less than half of normal." In the second patient, an electrocardiographic examination revealed "a typical digitalis effect." These two non-fatal cases are considered by Dr. Henry as the most important evidence suggesting that the six deaths were caused by the fatal interaction he suspected, "digitalis toxicity occurring because of potassium deficit."

This is the way Dr. Henry believes the interaction works: the amphetamines produce a pathological loss of appetite (anorexia) which automatically reduces potassium intake. Loss of the body's store of potassium occurred because of the laxatives and thiazide diuretics being taken at the same time. Nuts, fruits, beans, leafy green vegetables—any of these could have helped to supply needed potassium, if appetite had been sufficient or if the patient had known what was happening. "The net result," Dr. Henry explained, "was a large deficit in intracellular and extracellular potassium." When the potassium level decreases, the muscle substance of the heart becomes sensitive to digitalis, and doses of digitalis which would ordinarily be nontoxic become toxic. Dr. Henry concluded, "In summary, it would seem that the rainbow pills are dangerous and potentially fatal because of their propensity for causing potassium deficit and digitalis intoxication . . ."

Reports of fatalities kept appearing despite the repeated warnings and the publicity. The death of a nineteen-year-old boy was reported in the 1969 *Journal of the American Medical Association*. He entered the Neurological Service of the Los Angeles County-University of Southern California Medical Center complaining of progressive weakness of two days' duration. It took a few hours for doctors treating him to discover what medications he had been taking, specifically diet drugs, whereupon they began potassium therapy given intravenously. By that time it was too late for the boy's body to benefit from the potassium. Despite cardioversion and cardiac massage, he died thirteen hours after being admitted to the Center.

His history is typical of diet drug deaths. In January 1967, he was in good health, except for his obesity; he weighed 300 pounds. After a visit to the same doctor who was treating his mother, also for obesity, the boy received prescriptions for a thyroid preparation, digitalis, amphetamines, potassium gluconate, and chlorthalidone. He soon began to lose weight, and, by September of that same year, although complaining of "aching joints," the youth had lost 70 pounds and was feeling "essentially well." The last time he saw his diet doctor, his dose of potassium was increased to one gram daily, in response to the boy's complaints of aches and pains. Obviously it was a case of too little, too late, because eleven days later he was dead.

Postmortem chemical studies revealed digitalis in the myocardium and amphetamines in the liver. Failure of the autopsy to show any other cause of death led the doctors who reported his case to the *Journal* to believe death was "due to the combined effect of weight control medications causing myocardial irritability, cardiac arrhythmias, and hypokalemia." It was the conclusion of this report that obesity alone is not a valid reason for large doses of thyroid, digitalis, and "prolonged fluid depletion by long-term diuretic administration."

Drs. Jelliffe, Hill, Tatter, and Lewis, authors of the article, have this to say about diet medication: "this case represents a death due to the total effect of all the medications he received for weight reduction. It is quite possible, however, that each medication, if taken by itself in similar doses, probably would not have caused death . . . There is no universally safe and effective therapy for obesity."

The era of blind reliance on doctors to administer safe combinations of drugs has to be over with the "rainbow pill story." Patients are going to have to ask what they are being given and to learn just what those long Latin words mean in terms of their effect on the body.

The Pep-Pill Generation

Amphetamines in high doses affect the behavior of the individual so that he has difficulty functioning properly in his social environment. The user develops a tolerance followed by "an intense psychological dependence," explains Dr. George R. Edison in the April 1971 issue of the *Annals of Internal Medicine*. That means, whatever dose a person starts taking, he will probably increase it until changes in his behavior become apparent to those around him. According to Dr. Edison, in order to provide amphetamines in adequate supply "to treat the exceptional case in which the drug is truly indicated," we would need "less than one percent of the current volume of amphetamine production"! Dr. Edison calls the use of amphetamines "perhaps the most serious drug abuse" excepting in large cities where heroin addiction is widespread. (In those cities, amphetamines may be a close second.)

Why are such dangerous drugs still used so readily? Dr. Edison believes that most doctors feel the need to offer something to the patient trying to lose weight. The economic value of sales of the drug is substantial, judging from the industry's enthusiastic promotion of these drugs and tens of thousands of respectable adults who are to some extent dependent on them and persuade their doctors to keep prescribing them. Dr. Edison also thinks that doctors themselves use and abuse psychoactive drugs more often than the general public, thereby having some trouble evaluating the use of these drugs for their patients. (All the more reason for the layman to do some evaluating on his own!)

Amphetamine production in the United States in

1971 was sufficient to supply 40 doses for every man, woman, and child in this country annually. Not only do the obese become addicted to these temporary "lifters," but many truck drivers take them to stay awake during those long hauls on the road, and many college students "pop uppers" to stay awake all night and cram for exams. Even some athletes take them to gain artificial energy. Serious physical harm ultimately results for athletes who come to depend on the "pep pills" because they mask symptoms of fatigue, forcing already overworked bodies to work even harder. One rookie athlete tossed down six amphetamines at once; the result was convulsions and coma.

People who use amphetamines often find themselves in serious trouble before fully realizing what has happened. That "good feeling" brought on by the diet pill lasts only a few hours, and is often followed by depression and exhaustion. The temptation to take another pill is easy to give in to, and, once you get used to the timing, you can take one before the effect of the last one wears off. A vicious cycle is set into motion.

Some people can lose weight with them. Long-term users of amphetamines sometimes suffer from malnutrition becase they lack all desire to eat. In other people, the effect of appetite control soon wears off, but they keep taking the pill for the other feelings it promotes. They not only fail to lose significant amounts of weight, they've started themselves on a drug habit. With amphetamine addiction come the "bonuses" of headache, dehydration, dry mouth, cracked lips, bad breath, aggressiveness, irritability sometimes resulting in violence, and a rapid heartbeat that can cause heart block.

Other nations have their problems with amphetamines. Sweden eased the laws regulating their use in 1965, and in 1966 declared the move an unmitigated disaster. In Stockholm alone, users of amphetamines jumped from 3,000 to 6,000. Large numbers of people were being hospitalized with paranoid psychosis traced to use of the drug. The results were so alarming that Sweden banned amphetamines entirely. In 1971 they could not even be prescribed by a physician.

Switzerland, Austria, and West Germany also outlawed several types of amphetamines after discovering some link between them and heart rhythm disturbance.

What was happening to the drug in the United States in 1971? Some officials were becoming increasingly alarmed at the spreading amphetamine problem. Authorities were considering computerizing or tracking amphetamines from manufacturer to druggist to prescription in an effort to curb black market traffic. Many doctors were still recommending and prescribing this pill for dieting.

In 1972 the abuse of amphetamines was a major subject for two weeks testimony before the Subcommittee on Monopoly of the Senate Select Committee on Small Business, questioning whether manufacturers making the drug and doctors prescribing it ought to be told to stop. Dr. Henry E. Simmons, director of the Food and Drug Administration's Bureau of Drugs, testified that the agency would soon move to restrict further the power of doctors to prescribe amphetamines for weight reduction.

Doctors called to testify at the hearings used

"harsh terms" in accusing the public of "believing . . . myths about obesity, doctors of pandering to these misbeliefs, and drug companies of promulgating the distortions for profit," according to the *New York Times* reporter Richard D. Lyons.

Dr. Jean Mayer was there, opening fire not only on drugs but also on fad diets, branding concoctions like the rice diet and the-drinking-man's-diet extreme and even dangerous.

Dr. Thaddeus E. Prout, chief of medicine at the Greater Baltimore Medical Center, implied that drug companies, which "spend 12,000,000 dollars yearly to advertise in A.M.A. publications, had put pressure on the association and persuaded it to disband its Council on Drugs several months ago 'for reasons of economy'."

The doctors who testified found amphetamines relatively useless in the control of obesity, but despaired of turning doctors away from prescribing them or the public away from taking them in an effort to lose weight. They felt that most doctors were essentially bored with the problem of weight control, and diet pills were an easy way to "brush off" the patient. There was further testimony on the fact that there were a large number of fat people, which may be why they are so interesting to pharamaceutical manufacturers. The testimony was damning, but firm action against amphetamines was yet to be forthcoming.

Diet Drugs: the Loser's Game

In an evaluation of the role of diet drugs in the treatment of obesity, Dr. Herbert Gershberg of the New York School of Medicine, writing in *Postgraduate*

Medicine, May, 1972, says, "Many drugs have been used in attempts to promote weight loss. They include drugs producing anorexia, drugs causing nausea, drugs preventing gastrointestinal absorption, hormones increasing metabolism and lipolysis, tranquilizers, and diuretics. None has been shown in properly controlled investigations to be more effective than a placebo (a preparation containing no medicine but given for its psychological effect) when they are given in conjunction with a low-calorie diet."

Dr. Gershberg points out that when thyroid hormone is given to obese patients "in an office, clinic, or outpatient setting, as one to three grams of desiccated thyroid or its equivalent daily, it is not more effective than diet alone. Even nine grams daily does not consistently induce more weight loss than diet alone."

1972 also brought another warning, this time from the Better Business Bureau of Greater Philadelphia. The Bureau charged as untrue claims of advertisements that one could lose "seven pounds in 48 hours" and "up to 71 pounds in less than three months" without exercising, dieting, or using dangerous drugs." They referred to ads that "discuss the conversion of calories to energy rather than fat and imply that their pill will help metabolize calories into energy."

The B.B.B. exposed these pills as "a combination of benzocaine and a form of methylcellulose. Cellulose is often used in weight-reducing pills as a filler or bulk agent and is also found in some laxatives. Benzocaine is a local or topical anesthetic which may tend to dull the taste buds." It also may be remembered that cellulose acts as a laxative *instead of* a filler in most cases. The Bureau also pointed out that benzocaine is largely ineffective because appetite is based on factors other than taste.

Did this kind of information put our friends benzocaine and cellulose out of business? Currently, we can read in the Sunday paper's supplement of the miraculous "X-11." "EAT WELL . . . AND LOSE UGLY FAT. Lose 5, 10, 25 or More Pounds of Fat while you enjoy Eating Foods you buy in any grocery store. Get rid of Unsightly Bulges—ALL OVER! Contains one of the strongest diet aids available without prescription." Does this pitch sound familiar? The ad continues, "Take one of these tablets a half hour or so before your regular meals. It combines a pure vegetable extract that has no calories, and starts acting to provide a feeling of a fuller stomach. Satisfies appetite. Appeases taste-sense. Supplements vitamins."

In 1972, Senator Warren Magnuson introduced a bill to fire all F.D.A. bureaucrats, provide fines for company executives who knowingly endanger the public, permit citizens to sue lackadaisical government employees, and reorganize the whole Food and Drug Administration under the name of the Consumer Safety Agency. And what was going on back at the pharmaceutical companies? They were devoting major research efforts towards the creation of what they privately called a "pig pill." This pill is supposed to interfere with both digestion and absorption to the extent that you can develop a figure as graceful as a gazelle's while eating with the proverbial appetite of a hog. According to British zoologist Dr. Alex Comfort, writing in the *New Scientist,* this pill is bent on achieving for our age what the gluttonous Romans achieved when they stuck their fingers down their throats during a banquet in order to disgorge what they had already eaten and make room for the next stupendous course of the dinner.

The companies working on this pill may have obtained the idea from the "pig operation" which we have described earlier. That surgical procedure ran into trouble when one surgeon was having an especially hectic day—three pig operations scheduled! He snipped and stitched a patient's intestines the wrong way so that everything the poor fellow ate went *back into* his stomach, with fatal results.

Or the idea for the pig pill may have been inspired by some scientist watching a garbage disposal at work.

At any rate, this all-time longest-running horror show seemed to reach a climax in 1972. With the denouement of slowly awakening public awareness and the glimmers of congressional action, one would expect 1973 to be the "year of decision."

Apparently though, HCG, the sex hormone, was not only still being studied, but still being used in the treatment of obesity. One study admits that the controversy over human chorionic gonadotrophin goes on, but even though it's not safe and not completely understood as to its total effect, doctors are still submitting patients to its risks.

Drs. W. L. Asher and Harold W. Harper presented a report in the *American Journal of Clinical Nutrition,* February, 1973, from the American Society of Bariatric Physicians Research Council: "Effect of Human Chorionic Gonadotrophin on Weight Loss, Hunger, and Feeling of Well-Being." Dr. Harper "has an active practice using HCG in weight reduction." In the course of an experiment using HCG on one group and a placebo on another, while both groups were advised to follow the usual strict 500- to 550-calorie diet, it was found that the group having HCG shots lost a lot more weight, but, as the report states, "It seems unlikely that, if both groups had followed their diets strictly, there would have been a significant difference in weight loss between the groups."

The theory that evolved from this experiment seems to support Dr. Simeons' contention: that HCG is not responsible for weight reduction, but that, while on the low-calorie diet, it makes the patient less hungry and generally in better spirits. Extending the theory a bit further, under HCG therapy a patient would be more motivated to adhere to the starvation regimen because of the "lift" that the drug gave, while the person receiving the placebo wouldn't have that crutch to take his mind off hunger.

Later in the report there is this question raised: "Whether the long-term results of weight loss using single or multiple courses of HCG injections are better than the usual dismal long-term results of weight reduction needs objective examination. It seems doubtful such would be the case unless the physician involved continued to work vigorously with the patient in the re-education of eating patterns." The latter, of course, is what we've been proposing all along—learning new eating habits—but without the expensive (in more ways than one) HCG "trip," which would only delay the re-education process.

The accompanying starvation diet customarily used with HCG would springboard the patient back to old eating habits as soon as he was "free" of it. It is much more sensible and successful to adopt a moderate diet which is designed to be continued, with enjoyment, indefinitely. If the diet *can* be enjoyed, it has a much better chance of being continued.

Also in 1973, the *Journal of the American Medical Association* published a survey of United States physicians on "Attitudes toward Appetite Suppressants," by Dr. Louis Lasagna, Department of Pharmacology and Toxicology, University of Rochester School of Medicine and Dentistry, New York. One is surprised that this is still an unsettled question, but Dr. Lasagna's opening remarks are concise and illustrative of the situation as it existed at the time of the survey: "The use of anorexigenic drugs in medicine is a controversial subject. The traditional academic line has described the amphetamines and newer compounds as drugs of limited utility, with a weak initial effect to which tolerance develops rapidly, and with a considerable potential for inducing a psychologic dependence. This attitude contrasts sharply with the national sales figures of appetite suppressants, which indicate a considerable prescribing of such agents by physicians."

Because law enforcement agencies were concerned about the production and "a possible major diversion" of these drugs into illicit channels of distribution, amphetamine manufacturers were ordered to limit their 1972 production to "less than 18 percent of the 1971 figures."

Of the 686 doctors contacted, 70 percent granted complete interviews. Most of the doctors polled, the report stated, see and treat "a significant number" of obese patients each month. To the question what percentage of patients were currently being treated with appetite suppressants, Dr. Lasagna reported, 22 percent of the general practitioners, 43 percent of the obstetrician-gynecologists group, and 50 percent of the internists said they did not prescribe any appetite suppressants. "The others varied greatly in the frequency with which they prescribe such drugs."

When the 172 doctors who said they did not use anorexiants were asked why, 34 percent considered the drugs ineffective, 15 percent said the effects were temporary and the patients regained the lost weight, and 27 percent just "didn't believe in" using appetite suppressants.

About 25 percent of the physicians "feared addiction or dependency, 20 percent preferred their patients to exercise or to rely on diet. Seven percent admitted that the drugs are dangerous, 11 percent of the obstetricians said they were unsafe during pregnancy, 3 percent said they were contraindicated in patients with cardiac disease, 3 percent said they produced unpleasant side effects." Only 3 percent said they did not use them because of legal restrictions (If you're a rapid math freak and have come up with a total like 148 percent, Dr. Lasagna explained that's "because of multiple reasons being given by some respondents."

The names of the drugs that were used most popularly by the doctors who favored them were: Tenuate (diethylpropion), then Preludin (phenmetrazine hydrochloride). Next in order: Eskatrol (a dextroamphetamine sulfate and prochlorperazine maleate combination), Dexamyl (a dextroamphetamine sulfate and amobarbital combination), Ionamin (phentermine resin), Pre-Sate (chlorphentermine hydrochloride),

Tepanil (diethylpropion hydrochloride), Dexedrine (dextroamphetamine sulfate), Biphetamine (dextroamphetamine and amphetamine combination), amphetamine, Obedrin (methamphetamine hydrochloride/ pentobarbital/ ascorbic acid/ thiamine mononitrate/ niacin/ riboflavin combination (Good grief!), Desbutal (methamphetamine hydrochloride and pentobarbital sodium combination), Plegine (phendimetrazine tartrate), dextroamphetamine, Didrex (benzphetamine hydrochloride), and the mixtures of dextroamphetamine sulfate and meprobamate—Appetrol and Bamadex.

Dr. Lasagna remarked that a significant number of the physicians expressed expectations about the rate at which their patients would lose weight while on these drugs, "that seem likely to be doomed to disappointments even with patients who adhere rigidly to diets."

The physicians using the drugs in their treatment of obese patients assessed the efficacy of the drugs as follows: seven percent said "excellent," 24 percent thought they were "good," 42 percent only rated them "fair," and 27 percent admitted to "poor." The question arises, why were the doctors who rated amphetamines for appetite control "fair" or "poor" still using them on patients, having once made this low value judgment? You have probably already noted that this was by far the larger percentage.

What about side effects? 28 percent of the prescribing doctors mentioned no troublesome side effects or problems, 39 percent noted stimulation or overstimulation in their patients using the drugs, 22 percent mentioned dependency, 21 percent noted insomnia, three percent saw elevated blood pressure, three percent recorded depression in their patients taking amphetamines, and two percent noticed nausea or gastric upset.

The question of the potential abuse of the drugs by their patients was answered by the doctors rather vaguely or with the use of hedging modifiers. But the doctors had no hesitation in projecting that the abuse potential in drugs obtained from illicit sources might be great. The danger was rated at the highest possible level by 73 percent. Still trying to fathom the complexities of these doctors' logic, the questionnaire asked if appetite suppressants, because they are subject to abuse by users, should be removed from the market. One percent expressed no opinion, 30 percent of the doctors said "no," and 69 percent surprised us with a "yes." Of the 135 who thought appetite suppressants should be banned, 45 percent wanted that whole class of drug taken off the market, 38 percent just wanted amphetamines removed, 10 percent mentioned others, and seven percent didn't commit themselves.

The two most popular drugs in use, Tenuate and Preludin, have been demonstrated for several years to be ineffective in the treatment of obesity, notably by Modell in 1960 and Fazekas in 1961. Preludin was named by two British doctors in 1962 as a possible cause of abnormal births. In Spain and Germany, the manufacturers of this reducing drug warned against its use during pregnancy; in Italy, it was withdrawn from the market at once.

At the same time, in the United States, the government took no action at all, and the U. S. producers of Preludin denied there could be any danger in their product. One wonders if doctors in America were so busy with large practices that they had no time to read medical literature on the subject of these drugs.

That the prescription of reducing drugs is lucrative for manufacturers and physicians is obvious by now. With so much eye-closing and foot-dragging in the past on the part of regulatory and law enforcement agencies in this field, one finds it difficult to place confidence in recent attempts at control of this situation.

The April 3, 1973 edition of the *Washington Post* reported that the federal government "will recall diet drugs that contain amphetamines because it says some are unsafe and some do not contribute to weight loss." In 1973, 480 million dosage units were being sold annually, according to a government spokesman. This would make it "the largest recall ever made of controlled substances." June 30 was set as the target date to remove "injectable amphetamines and amphetamines combined with such things as sedatives, tranquilizers, and vitamins." The action was based on the F.D.A.'s conclusion (finally) that the "injectable form is unsafe and that all the ingredients in the various products do not contribute to the claimed weight loss."

At this point, four of the firms involved asked for a hearing with the F.D.A. for five combination products. Naturally, these drugs would remain on the market until the matter was settled. Also, some of the diet drugs being used were not listed with the ones being removed from the market.

Still, it's a victory of sorts, at long last. A further irony lies in the fact that, while the government took more than a decade to make up its mind about diet drugs, it was nevertheless able to mount an all-out attack in short order against certain vitamins on grounds that are, at least, questionable.

While many of the fantastic lengths to which peo-ple will go in order to lose weight (while steadfastly resisting all sensible means) are amusing when viewed objectively, there is nothing funny about a kind of Medical Mafiosa of "fat doctors" dispensing useless or dangerous drugs profusely, and reaping enormous profit from short visits and sure-to-repeat clientele. We have gone into detail in naming these drugs and out-lining their supposed effect, as opposed to their real effects and side-effects, in the hope of making dieters more aware of the frustrations and dangers involved. Hopefully, the same critical assessment may be applied to any future drug recommended by a doctor or ad-vertised in glowing terms in a magazine.

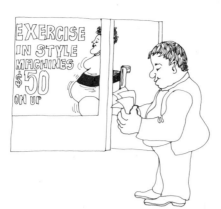

"Go for Broke"—Buy Expensive Reducing Equipment

If you're really "into" the automated, technical age and don't want to change your starchy-sugary hangup, there are misguided faddists and self-guided hucksters ready to help you with a host of shiny, elaborate equipment for keeping fit. Of course, the machines will do the work, and there will be no effort required on your part—that's what makes the program so difficult to resist!

Exercise *is* essential to having a trim, fit body, and some exercises are sensible and beneficial. All of these require effort, but it can be quite enjoyable. Increased physical activity is half the battle of the bulge; a reasonable, healthful diet is the other half.

But, out in the wonderful world of free enterprise, there are any number of handsome, muscular men and scantily-clad, shapely women ready to sell you an "easy way" to tone up your body and lose weight without tiresome activity or restrictive diets. If your ego is sagging with your belly and your favorite hobby is wasting money, you'll find something there to oblige every preference.

Abdominal belts, elastic abdominal belts, and sauna belts are currently fashionable for re-capturing the slim waist of one's youth. If no effort is required in using the equipment, other than that of writing a check, no benefit will result except a temporary squeezing of flesh not unlike what happens to your arm if you put an elastic band around it. As you know, the indentation is gone soon after the elastic is removed.

If the belt you are considering does require that you exercise (way down in the small print of the ad) and then suggests that you wear the belt so that "it can do its work while you do whatever you like," the *exercise* is the real agent of change. If you threw away the belt and just did the exercise, you would accomplish the same amount of waist-trimming. The belt, an advertisement declares, is to "make your body heat sweat away the excess moisture that adds to bulky fat"—which is just a fancy way of saying you'll lose water from the tissue but not fat. It is the fat you must lose if you are obese.

Robert Sherrill, in a report in *Today's Health,* August 1971, pointed out that in *1950* an elastic abdominal belt was ruled off the market for fraudulent advertising by its promoters. Far from discouraging the buying public, these early skirmishes with the law have been largely ignored by gullible fatties. Of course, in any circumstances where a promoter is constrained from selling his product because of false claims—and even when prosecuted—it's a simple matter for him to launch another (strangely similar) product from another locale, or sell the company to a relative, or change the name of the product and start selling it again.

The sauna belt is the latest version of the reducing belt, but it differs little from the earlier versions. It is inflated before exercising and left on for a time after exercising to allow your midsection to "steam." The manufacturers voice the usual "guarantee," but the Post Office and 14,000 customers have already complained, because the belt won't do anything for you that exercising alone won't do. Federal examiners have also warned that the belt can prove harmful and that it is not really a new device.

Cleanliness may be next to Godliness, but it will do nothing for your weight. Nevertheless, at least 700 people bought Formula XR-6, a bath additive that was supposed to take 61 pounds off the purchaser if he put 2 cupfuls in his bath for five baths in a row.

As if you don't have enough to worry about if you're fat, there's a new wrinkle called "cellulite," which is supposed to be an even uglier kind of fat than ordinary fat. "WHAT IS CELLULITE?" asks the advertisement for Mme. Nicole Ronsard's book *Cellulite: Those Lumps Bumps and Bulges You Couldn't Lose Before,* sold at a whopping $12.95 per copy, and it continues in fine print, "Don't let the word frighten you." (Already you're frightened enough to be looking in the mirror with alarm.) "Millions of women everywhere have cellulite and live their lives with it . . . simply because they have never been able to recognize it, and thus have not been able to do anything about it. Now, thanks to the efforts of Mme. Ronsard, the prayers of many can be answered."

The reader of this ad is not going to be one of those lucky women who lived with cellulite and never even knew they were blighted, because the text goes on to explain in detail "unslightly lumps and bulges" that are "more than simple fatty tissue. It is a gel-like substance made up of fat, water, and wastes trapped in immovable pockets beneath the skin."

There *is* hope, however. "Say good-bye to 'jodhpur thighs' and saddlebag buttocks' . . . never again be embarrassed by 'cottage cheese' textured skin . . . To discover if you have a cellulite problem, take one simple test that cannot fail: Squeeze the tissues between the thumb and index finger or between the palms of both hands. If cellulite is present, skin ripples and looks like an orange peel. At a more advanced stage, ripples will be noticeable without any pressure." Is there a gal who won't try this test immediately?

If you really want to know more about cellulite without spending $12.95 to learn about a problem you never knew you had, the November, 1973 issue of *Playgirl* had an article in it about cellulite, with the provocative lead-in "The French Have a Word for It . . ." Cellulite, it explained, is the French word for fibrositis, an inflammation of the fibrous tissue, which may go hand in hand with circulatory troubles. Improper elimination and not drinking enough water to allow the kidneys to do their job of flushing out the toxins are cited as causes by M. Jane Campbell, author of the report, plus many of the evils of our modern life, such as "tension, lack of exercise, inability to relax and sleep, hasty eating habits, improper diet laced with food additives and chemicals."

Proper diet, elimination of coffee and alcohol, reduction of starch, sugar, and salt intake, and drinking plenty of fresh water are self-help methods suggested by the article, along with deep stroking massage.

Looking beautiful is a prime motivation in our society, and good health runs second, as every entrepreneur of the fitness game knows. Interestingly enough, it's in the beauty area that exploiters get a chance to work the other side of the street: not only can you make some too-large parts of you smaller, but you can make the too-small parts of you bigger. We are indebted again to the Guinness Book of World Records for the information that the smallest waist on an adult woman ever recorded was only thirteen inches.

Newspapers and magazines which are oriented toward a female readership frequently carry advertisements for various kinds of "bust developers." The "pitch" is to make you self-conscious about the size of your bust, if you are built on a small scale, without any regard to the aesthetics of proportion.

"My Bustline increased from 36 inches to a Full 40 inches in just 6 weeks" reads the text under a startling caption: "Mark Eden is the World's most successful bustline developer." For just $9.95, the company will ship you an "exerciser that employs special techniques" with a kit that includes the "Contouring Course"—all in a plain wrapper, so that the postman will not leer at you.

Then there's the "Beauty Persuader"—$9.98 with a "guide" and "complete plan"—which will "build a beautiful bustline in just 5 minutes a day . . . via unique extension-contraction principle."

There are other companies, of course, which promise more or less the same amazing results; their glowing advertisements are illustrated with "unretouched" photographs of young ladies with such astonishing busts ("after" buying the "plan") that one wonders if they can sit up without help. These back-of-the-magazine offers appear to flourish through all the erratic vogues in figure, even when fashion dictates the "flat look."

Actually, the size of one's bustline cannot be increased, but the bust can be made more shapely in a way that appears fuller by proper exercise. Exercise plans are available in many books and magazines; there's no need to send for any special equipment or kit.

Then there's the business of "body shaping." The "5 minute total body-shaper and slimming course" (again in a plain wrapper for a modest $9.95) promises "amazing results in just 3 days!" Here's what you get, and, indeed, it seems to be quite a bargain: the course "reshapes your legs to more pleasing lines . . . slenderizes, tightens up your hiplines . . . slims 3 inches in 7 days off your waistline . . . reduces protruding tummy in just 7 days . . . firms, uplifts, shapes your total bustline . . . firms up shoulders, chin, neckline, arms, as well as enhancing body posture and realigning figure beauty" with this "ingenious 16-ounce Body Shaper . . . Without giving up the foods you love!"

The ad makes sport of other fads, including belts, shorts, and so forth, and, having noted the fakes that appeal to your laziness, explains that you achieve these fantastic improvements by "doing one simple 5 minute continuous rhythm-coordinated exercise, lying on your back!"

In another ad, the "16-ounce Body Shaper" becomes the "1 pound Waist Slimmer." This, too, takes only 5 minutes each day, and the texts are basically the same in both advertisements, although slightly re-arranged; the price of the "Slimmer," like the "Shaper," is $9.95. Oh yes, and the address you send to get it is the same in both cases, also.

In case your busy social schedule just doesn't give you that all-important 5 minutes a day, the "Slumber-Shapers, Inc." of Miami, Florida, has a "remarkable break-through in weight reduction" to help you out. With a "new miracle fabric" called "Isosaunatrex" you "Reduce While You Sleep"—"no strenuous exercises—no special diets." These "Slumber-Shapers" massage away fatty tissue with the slightest movement of your body." You may also be comforted by the knowledge that they're virtually indestructible, flame-resistant, and won't mildew . . . completely washable and rapid drying." In addition to the $1.00 to cover postage and handling, and another $1.00 if you can't wait and want your order rushed, you merely send $14.98 for the "Long Line" or $11.98 for the "Short Line" or $9.98 if you just want a couple of things to slip around your thighs.

By the way, the kit *does* include "a supplemental exercise booklet, and diet plan," which is interesting when you consider that the Slumber-Shaper is supposed to work while you're asleep. We would venture to guess that the kit works a lot better if you do exercise and diet. In fact, perhaps you could manage to get along with exercise and diet alone, and save a little money toward your new wardrobe!

Body Persuasion System, Inc., manufactures a series of "helpers" listed by Aileen Jacobson in the *Washington Post's* magazine section Potomac, July, 1973. (The Postal Service has instituted formal proceedings against B.P.S., Inc.) The items include Slimmers, Glove ("lick the globbies and stay globbie-free all your life"), Isotensor Bustline Increasor, and Beauty Breast of Paris, "a cup-like device that sprays water, which Gene McHale, an investigator in the U.S. Postal Service, described as a Rube Goldberg machine," comments Miss Jacobson.

If all of this seems female-oriented, don't think that the vanity market that men represent is overlooked. For only $7.99 they can have the Jay Norris Corp. of Freeport, New York, send them what looks very much like a girdle. Under the trade name of "Tru-Health," these briefs provide "super control that *really* slims you!" And this miracle, of course, happens "instantly."

Hanover House of Hanover, Pennsylvania offers for $9.98, plus 75¢ for postage and handling, an "amazing simple two-step program" that will reduce not only your neck wrinkles but also your double chin. This "Magic Mold Home Anatone" program combines the use of a "special formula cream . . . massage" and a "magic-like Syncromesh Spandex" mold you put over your chin(s). According to the accompanying illustration, it also covers your upper neck and crosses over the top of your head (giving you that Knight Errant look) for "45 minutes at a time."

Having noted all these "amazing" or "magic" results from wrapping various parts of your body and head, doesn't it make sense to believe you can achieve positive miracles by wrapping your entire frame in the style of an Egyptian mummy? Whether the plan is packaged under the name "Insta-Trim," "Suddenly-Slenda," "Suddenly-Slim," "Swiss-Trim," "Benne Method," "Body Wrap," "Shape Wrap," "Continental Miracle Wrap," or "Figure Wrap," the advertisements invariably promise three to 15 inches off certain strategic locations in an hour, in a week, or somewhere between.

Since the charge ranges from $25.00 to $150.00 for the treatments, you might like to know what you get for your money. First of all, they measure you, undressed, and you'd better check on the way they hold that tape measure. Then your entire body is wrapped in "glamour tapes" which have been soaked in a "magical solution." The tapes are Ace bandages or the equivalent, and, usually, the magic solution is Epsom salts and alum. Next you slip into a rubberized sauna suit that fits tightly around ankles and wrists. Your attendants make you as comfortable as possible under the circumstances for about an hour, often tucking a cosy, warm blanket over your suit. When the time's up, you're measured again, and, lo and behold, the miracle has occurred. You've been dehydrated and indented, and, with the tape measure pulled *tightly* this time, you are inches slimmer. With such marvelous results achieved in such a short time, wouldn't you want to sign up for the whole series of 20 sessions?

This isn't a new "con"—it's been going on for several years. The names keep changing to give you the feeling that a new discovery has been made, but what you've actually paid for is temporary dehydration. If you'd really like to challenge one of these outfits, insist they measure you again a few days later to see if you have maintained the "loss." Even a few hours later should see the return of fluid to your tissues.

The temporary shrinking of your body, which is much slighter than it seems, due to the deftness of the "before" and "after" measurers, is also the result of an indentation which any tight wrapping, such as a belt or a girdle, will produce in your flesh. This may give you a smaller waist, but the pressure of the tapes may have also reduced the amount of blood in the body's surfaces, diverting it into deeper body tissue as well as into the internal organs.

Body wrapping can also cause changes in your temperature, pulse, blood pressure, and respiration—as would happen if you were exposed to dehydration due to heat exhaustion. After all, you have inhibited the radiation of heat from your skin by allowing yourself to be encased in a tape-and-rubber cocoon for an hour or more. The magnesium sulphate may produce irritation and softening of the tissues, and you could develop a heat rash from the anti-perspirant action of the aluminum sulphate.

There are other "magic solutions" which can bring about a temporary shrinkage. These "secret formulas" could be glycerine, which absorbs moisture from the body and could dehydrate the superficial tissues, or even common table salt, in sufficient concentration, which can produce a hypertonic effect—that is, reduce the fluid content of the blood stream over the entire body through the exertion of an osmotic pressure.

Then there's always the action of hypothermy.

Is the salon air-conditioned? Of course. Once the blanket's gone, the suit and bandages off, and there you are, soaked in sweat, the cool air that hits your body produces a constriction of the surface blood vessels. If you are measured without delay, that constriction will reveal itself in a reduction of the size of your body parts.

Science has not yet invented a chemical substance that will cause a permanent reducing effect or melt fat away when applied to the body's surface. If you buy such a service, you will, at best, have wasted your money—at worst, caused yourself discomfort, if not damage, by the abuse of heat and cold and pressure. The fat your body stores is housed in "fat cells," and there's no way it can be "drawn out through your pores" while you sweat heavily. You can't sweat it out —nor can you push it, squeeze it, or shake it out.

One "magic formula" was described by the distributor as "100 percent protein natural organic formula." On analysis, it turned out to be less than one percent protein. (Windsor House, Island Park, Long Island, New York: wrap and solution: $7.99). Another solution called "special slim wrap formula" proved to be 99 percent Epsom Salts (Harvest House, Farmingdale, Long Island, New York: wrap and solution: $9.98). The price of Epsom Salts, as you probably know, is considerably less when purchased under its own name.

It is important to note that body wraps are potentially dangerous for people afflicted with diabetes or diseases of the arteries and veins of the extremities.

The "Benne Method" not only employs soaked tapes but also adds the bonus of massage, plus the aura of a celebrity clientele—Jane Fonda, as well as Robert Horton, and other Hollywood and T.V. personalities, models, executives, and so forth, have used this method of gilding the lily. Whatever your figure problem—heavy thighs, midriff bulge, double chin, upper arm sag—New York's Ben Benne will "re-shape" you by taping, manipulating, and pounding until your contours are changed to your satisfaction. The secret 5-chemical solution used to soak the tapes is, Benne says, "so non-toxic you can drink it."

This program is designed primarily as a "reconstruction" job which promises that it will cause unsightly fat to disappear from wherever it lumps and bumps to the surface, but it is doubtful that it is any different from the rest—in other words, if you exercise as part of the program, you will be helping your body to be more trim. For the rest of the "window dressing"—a series of ten treatments—it will cost you $110.00. And business is very good!

Sauna Treatments Are "Hot Stuff"

Like the belts and wraps, sauna shorts or the equivalent promise the disappearance of inches from hips, thighs, and waistlines—price from $4.00 to $13.00 per pair. You also receive a regimen of exercises. After working up a sweat with these, you put on the shorts so that your body heat will not be "allowed to escape." This is supposed to work "magic" on your figure, but, again, any magic here is in the exercises themselves.

In some cases, the shrinkage caused by the shorts shows up as expansion elsewhere. One man lost—

temporarily—three inches from his waist and gained three inches on his thighs, after following the exercise and shorts procedure. Another man, using the same program, lost an inch on his hips, put a half-inch *on* his waist, and added an inch and three-quarters to his thighs. A young woman, who did the same exercises as the two men but did not use the shorts, lost three-quarters of an inch from her waist and hips and two inches and three-quarters from her thighs, which may be informative to anyone who wishes to trim away inches while saving the price of unnecessary equipment.

Sauna suits, sometimes known as "trim jeans," are all more or less designed like gym suits—sweat shirts and sweat pants with elastic cuffs around wrists and ankles, elastic or draw-string around the waist, and snug fit around the neck. The basic idea is to hold in the body heat as you sweat from exercising. Slim-Ez Suit Co., Inc., of Chattanooga, Tennessee, manufactures one called "Trim-Ez" for $9.95. According to the promotional information, it "holds in body heat to lose weight faster while doing yardwork, housework, and exercise . . . acts as a steam bath to speed body conditioning as you bend or stretch with work or exercise. Trim down and tone muscles faster with much less effort. The rubberized miracle material is soft, lightweight, and comfortable . . . For fewer pounds and trimmer figure easier."

Imagine, for a moment, that your body is an engine with a thermostat. The "human thermostat" cannot be turned off to accommodate unnatural conditions, like wearing a sauna suit. Your body produces heat in many ways—by cell activity, muscle activity, food digestion, and hormone production. Your body also picks up heat from the sun or from its rays bounced off sand or snow. To protect itself from accumulating too much heat, your body sweats—losing heat through the skin's pores. (It also gets rid of excess heat through the lungs and through waste.) While exercising, the body's sweat is designed to keep it cool.

To shed heat from your body, the sweat must evaporate. Letting it run off you or wiping it off does nothing to make you cooler. Evaporation, on the other hand, cools the blood close to the surface of the skin, enabling that blood to return to the deeper "core tissues" inside your body. At the same time, the blood from those core tissues circulates toward your skin to continue the complete cooling process. Circulation is speeded up so that the heat exchange operates more efficiently. In other words, for sweat to perform its natural function—to act as a coolant—it must have a chance to evaporate adequately. In dry air, when it's warm with low humidity, the sweat will evaporate rapidly from the surfaces of the body. When there's a breeze, air currents contribute to a quicker cooling process. But what happens when it's warm and the humidity is high? The air is saturated with water and cannot absorb your sweat, which simply drips off your body. Not only is the blood near your skin not cooled, but there is no lowering of the temperature of your core tissues.

What you're really doing when you wear a sauna suit is creating an environment for your body that is warm and highly humid. The rubberized sweat suit does not allow the skin of your body to be exposed to air. It "traps" the heat your body gives off, and sweat cannot evaporate.

In creating such an environment, you may be inviting heat exhaustion. A sudden exposure to high temperatures will make the blood rush toward the surface of the body in an effort to carry the core heat to the skin where sweating can cool it through evaporation. The blood pressure drops as the blood reaches the surface capillaries. Blood volume is reduced, meanwhile, because some of the fluid passes into cells and evaporates as sweat. As the heart becomes less able to maintain blood pressure, circulation slows down. The core heat no longer escapes your body, and heat exhaustion can occur.

Signs to watch out for are profuse sweat, moist skin, rapid pulse, accompanied by great discomfort and gasping for breath. These symptoms precede collapse and unconsciousness from heat exhaustion. First aid treatment for this condition includes immediate reduction of the body temperature, plenty of fluids, and rest.

Another condition to watch out for is dehydration exhaustion—which can happen when you're not getting enough water while exercising. After all, your body is a delicately balanced mechanism. If you exercise strenuously, your body can lose over eight quarts of water in an hour and a half! In average exercise, a person normally sheds about three quarts of water in that amount of time. Since it's almost impossible to replace that much water in such a short time, your blood volume decreases and a stimulus is sent to the hypothalamus in your brain. The hypothalamus in turn sends signals for a hormone to be released which slows down the production of urine, for the sake of conserving the body's water supply. If heavy sweating continues and the fluid lost is not replaced, you can suffer heat stroke, a condition that spells real trouble and demands emergency action. (You may have heard of this kind of attack under the name "sunstroke.")

Heat stroke begins with a rising skin temperature, followed by sweating and expansion of the blood vessels. As the temperature goes up, there is even further expansion of the blood vessels, called vasodilation, and more sweating. Then sweating "efficiency" starts to decrease. When that occurs, the blood is no longer cooled adequately and the temperature of the core tissues rises. Sweating stops altogether, and a very dry skin results along with rising temperature—these are the chief symptoms of the onset of heat stroke. If the temperature is not reduced immediately, the cells of the brain can be permanently damaged. In some cases of "sunstroke," the victims die. Of course, conditions have to be extreme for this to happen, but it is wise to keep in mind the way in which the body works when exercising. Remember that it needs to sweat and it needs to replace the fluids it loses. Be especially careful when the humidity is high or when your body's subjected to the imposed humidity of a sauna.

Sauna baths, both commercial and "home portable," are very fashionable right now. Just to mention casually that you need the relaxation of a sauna after a hard day at the office implies that you are pressed by many executive responsibilities. In case you're a student of status symbols, having your own sauna at home has a little more *éclat* than having to stop at a health club.

As far back as the summer of 1970, the Federal Trade Commission warned the public of the potential dangers of sauna and steam baths. A preliminary investigation revealed that medical authorities had serious reservations about the medically unsupervised use of dry sauna or wet steam bath heat by untrained persons. Either kind of heat raises body temperature (hyperthermia) and blood pressure, and increases pulse rate. Older people and persons with diabetes, heart trouble, or high blood pressure may suffer harmful effects by taking sauna or steam baths. A physician's advice and guidance are essential under such circumstances. Adverse effects are also possible if one uses a steam or sauna bath within an hour after having eaten a heavy meal, or while under the influence of alcohol or drugs such as anticoagulants, antihistamines, vasoconstrictors, vasodilators, stimulants, hypnotics, narcotics, and tranquilizers.

Drs. Antonio Fornoza and Carlos Gutierre Salgado evaluated the effect of the sauna on the leukocytes (white blood cells) not so long ago, and their conclusion was that the sauna was stressful, physically, because it causes an increased secretion of hormones. They also noted that there's an individual difference among people in regard to their tolerance to heat. They recommended rigid medical control when using a sauna.

In another study, M. Huikko, P. Jouppila, and N. T. Karki reported that the sauna produces major changes in the circulatory system. Spending 30 to 60 minutes in a sauna can cause body temperature to rise as much as three degrees. Blood vessels dilate and peripheral resistance falls significantly. Cardiac output increases 73 percent and the pulse rate 61 percent. Systolic and diastolic blood pressures, however, remain practically unchanged, according to this report. Remaining in a sauna for long periods of time makes your body begin to absorb and store the heat, and this, as we have already observed, can lead to heat stroke. The three experts also mention the danger of dehydration, when the sweat loss can adversely affect the body, causing heat exhaustion. Authorities are not in agreement as to whether or not it is better to drink plenty of liquids before entering a sauna—but they are in agreement that only water weight is lost from sauna treatment and that the sauna in itself will not help to develop physical fitness.

If you're determined to buy a sauna anyway, it's not the time to try to save a few dollars on a "bargain." Some of them lack adequate safety devices and controls to prevent a prolonged, involuntary stay in the contraption in case of an accident. Some sauna and steam baths don't even include thermostats as standard equipment—they could become dangerously hot without your being aware of it!

Those portable steam cabinets which look like a black box—from which only your head protrudes while, inside, your body is being steamed—might be considered an invention of the devil. Nevertheless, in the illustration that accompanies the advertisement, the girl model, her hair wrapped in a towel and her imprisonment reminiscent of a magician's assistant in an infernal cabinet on stage, smiles blissfully to impress you with the beneficial effects she is enjoying.

At any rate, whichever you decide to purchase, "wet" or "dry," be certain that it has proper safety controls and a thermostat on which you can depend. Remember, too, that it may provide relaxation, if your physical health is good, but the one thing it will not do, no matter what the promotional material says, is to melt the fat off your body. Water, yes,—fat, no.

Shake, Rattle, and Roll Your Way to a New Figure

If you're really going to be up-to-date, perhaps the thing to do is to go electronic. True, there's an energy crisis and we should all try to conserve power, but the temptations of achieving a new figure without any effort on your part are very great. All you have to do is flip the switches! Maybe you don't have time for walking, jogging, bicycling, and swimming. Then, too, if you've attained a certain standing in your social circle, don't you owe it to yourself to own, if not the most expensive, certainly the latest weight-control gadget?

These are the psychological motivations which are taken into consideration, very seriously, by the promoters of machines which we never expected to see outside of a late night horror movie. If the "electronic muscle stimulator" makes you feel *too* stimulated as you lie there on your bed, you can switch to your "electronic muscle relaxer." Then you can get all tingly and refreshed by shaking in your automatic "belt massager," or, better yet, how about a "vibrating table"? Following up with an enlivening jolt from your portable "electric shock machine" should leave you ready for just about anything!

Of course, if there should be a power failure on

your block, you can have a "slimming wheel" tucked away in your closet for just such an emergency. You'll have to put a little effort into it, though. What you do with this gadget is to get on your knees, grasp the rod passed through the wheel's center with your hands, lean forward, and push the wheel back and forth on the floor. This is supposed to shrink your stomach from the first day you use it, according to Anthony Enterprises of San Francisco, California, who markets the device, called "Wonder Wheel." "A few rolls back and forth with Wonder Wheel from knee position equals 100 sit-ups." Right away, you know you're going to save a lot of time with this item. Some people take about three days to do 100 sit-ups—usually the very same individuals who are flipping through magazines looking for an easy way to become slim-hipped and muscular. The cost is a mere $3.98 plus 80¢ for mailing. Don't worry if you're the wobbly type (especially after a few drinks)—Anthony Enterprises manufactures a *double* wheel for the unskilled roller, for only $5.98 plus $1.00 mailing cost.

Once the electricity comes back on, you can go right back to something completely effortless, unless you're the nervous type. Remember the "Relaxacizor"? In 1970, the F.D.A. ruled that it could only be sold if prescribed by a doctor. (If you were farsighted enough, you'd already purchased yours anyway.) The Relaxacizor is an electric contrivance that sends current to your muscles through wires and contact pads strapped on your body. The electrical current forces your muscles to contract, and this is supposed to "firm up" the body and reduce your waistline. (The last time we saw something like this in action, Bela Lugosi was sending a charge through Boris Karloff.)

Unfortunately, it was potentially more than a few laughs. "In the hands of some 400,000 amateur and unsuspecting owners," said Robert Sherrill in the August, 1971 issue of *Today's Health,* "the Relaxacizor could, literally, be a death trap." The federal judge who issued the order halting the future sales of the machine, based on F.D.A. evidence, declared it was "capable of inducing heart failure" and could aggravate "gastrointestinal, orthopedic, muscular, neurological, vascular, dermatological, kidney, gynecological, and pelvic disorders." It might, he said, adversely influence conditions of "epilepsy, hernia, multiple sclerosis, spinal fusion, tubo-ovarian abuses, ulcers, and varicose veins" as well. The wonder is that the judge did not order the machines recalled and the money spent to purchase them refunded; if only part of this list of dangers were accurate, it would seem that further action was indicated.

The Relaxacizor first appeared on the market in 1949. In the 21 years during which it was available to the public (price range $100 to $1400), it is estimated to have grossed $40,000,000—and this "for a machine that the courts ultimately ruled not only worthless, but extremely dangerous." Why did it take so long to discover the machine's imperfections?

Hucksterism succeeds on the basis of a time-lag. It takes so long for government agencies to investigate, test, warn, build a case, and prosecute (not that the Government always wins the case, anyway) that the hucksters can become fabulously wealthy in the meantime. In the case of the Relaxacizor, the F.D.A. first forced the sellers to stop advertising that it would reduce weight, later to stop claiming it would reduce girth (the agile ad-writer is ever nimble, ever quick in jumping over one objectionable phrase and substituting another), and to desist from declaring that it would tone up muscles. "All this meant four or five years before we took them to court," Dr. Joe Davis of the F.D.A.'s office of evaluation of medical-clinical devices is quoted as saying, in Sherrill's report, "and after that we were in court for five or six more years."

The evidence provided by the sellers on the F.D.A.'s demand included about 1,000 complaints the company had received from customers, "and of these about 500 said they had been injured by the device," said Dr. Davis.

Is it a sufficient deterrent to force a product off the market and demand a fine (which, in contrast to the profits, may be negligible)? Wouldn't *realistic* fines and full restitution to the customers be more effective, especially in cases where fraud is compounded by the potential for harm, injury, or fatalities?

Another preventive measure might be to require "get-slim-quick-and-effortlessly" promoters to prove the safety and effectiveness of their devices before being permitted to offer them for sale. If this approach seems to be a harsh one, just keep in mind that winning the government's case against Relaxacizor cost the taxpayers a half million dollars!

Several variations of the "electric muscle stimulators" have been marketed, but basically they're much alike. This machine, neatly housed in a suitcase, offers an impressive array of dials and switches, and, of course, lots of wires with pads for attaching to parts of the body condemned to "reduction." The severity of the electrical charge can be regulated by turning the dials—all the way from a mild pinging sensation to a violent jolt (something like what you'd get a lot cheaper by sticking your finger into a live socket). The "shocked" muscles are supposed to contract and become "firmer, thereby reducing the size of the flabby areas."

Such artificially-induced contractions involve only local areas and not the whole body. They will not increase the body's metabolism, nor will they reduce anything but your patience. Ample curves and bulges will not disappear through the use of electric shock, because the body just doesn't dispose of fat in that manner. Actually, in the time it takes you to get rigged up in one of those contraptions, you could have been doing a number of *real* exercises to improve your figure—or you could have been jogging down to the bank to deposit the hundreds you saved by not buying ineffective machinery.

"Muscle tone" is a term that is often mentioned—in a nebulous way—in advertisements for this kind of equipment. What it really means is, the state of contraction of a muscle even when you're at rest. The degree of contraction depends on the response of the muscle to your nervous system. The stimulation it receives from the nervous system, whether one is standing up or lying down, determines the variation in tone. A claim of improved muscle tone made by promoters of electrical gadgets would prove difficult indeed to substantiate.

Nature has dealt many persons a little disproportion of face or figure—a heavy chin, large hips, or *something* that doesn't quite match the rest of them.

That's where "spot reducers" come into the profit picture! A spot reducer is any gadget you use to vibrate or to stimulate a particular part of your body—be it arm or leg or whatever. The important thing to remember is that there's no such thing as spot reducing—even exercise concentrated on one portion of your body will not make it less fatty than other portions. What exercise *will* do is to firm up the muscles in that area and to give the offending part a better appearance.

Fat reduction, when it occurs, happens all over the body, and exercise should be done with that in mind. Whatever is good for the whole body is good for its parts, also. It is impossible to redistribute fat, but it is possible to lessen it in an overall way. Once that is accomplished, an individual feels much more satisfied with himself and more able to accept gracefully the unique configurations of his frame. If one wants to do a little extra chin-stretching along with a regular program of total body exercise, that might be a good idea for firming up slackening muscles. But, if exercise won't do it, the job will certainly not be accomplished by a vibrating spot-reducing machine.

You may wonder about all those letters from satisfied users that appear in the advertisements of such gadgets. Enthusiastic testimonials, often with accompanying photographs, are used liberally throughout ads for the most astounding machines and equipment. If J. Doe of Oshkosh, Wisconsin, has found new beauty and confidence through the use of a particular contrivance, won't it be of benefit to you, too?

Assuming that the endorsements are not out-and-out phonies, composed by a desperate copywriter who only wants to make a living, it may be true that some people benefit from effortless exercising gadgets. Neurotic people often benefit in their imaginations when they try something new; they feel and look better to themselves *instantly,* which should be a clue. Manufacturers benefit, in dollars and cents. Well-known personalities benefit from the salaries paid to them for endorsing products which they have never used outside of the photograph studio.

There's no denying these kinds of benefits. What needs to be stressed though, is that the reader of an advertisement can never be quite sure just how these testimonials came about. Were they paid for by the company? Did the letter writer hope to receive at least a life-time supply of the product by writing a flattering endorsement? Is what appears in print an excerpt of the original letter? (Words like "amazing" and "fantastic" may have been taken from a sentence that read, "It's amazing how you crooks keep coming up with these fantastic swindles!")

Another thing to watch out for, in reading advertisements, is the misapplied logic. If a baseball team receives a free supply of some product, and many of the guys use it, then later that same team wins the pennant, does it necessarily follow that use of the particular product caused them to become champions? No testimonial from the team which *didn't* win *(who may have also been using the product)* will be solicited and paid for by the company.

What's in a name? "Health" Mattresses don't have any special features that make them more healthful than an ordinary good, firm mattress at ordinary prices. "Exercise" Sandals with wooden soles won't improve your physical fitness any more than ordinary sandals will. *Walking* is the thing that will really cause improvement. In fact, Exercise Sandals may give you tired legs.

Because of misleading advertising, the American public is being bilked out of $250 million annually for physical fitness. At least $100 million of this, according to the Wall Street Journal, results from the sale of "effortless" exercise equipment. Any advertisement that leads you to believe that "the machine will do it for you . . . ," that you can improve your figure without any activity on your part, should be highly suspect. If you really want to change the way you look and feel, to have a healthier, more vigorous body, you already own the best equipment in the world—two arms and two legs that can walk, swing, dance, swim, row, bicycle, and jog.

"How I Spent My Summer Vacation"

For many people, exercising alone at home, either with or without music-to-do-bends-and-lifts-by, is too boring a way to improve their figures. They like to be with other people, to enjoy the advice, admonishment, and praise of a trained exercise leader and to use the best gym equipment. It's relaxing and refreshing for individuals with high stress jobs to be catered to by professionals for a couple of hours a week.

Some overweight people just like a lot of personal attention; that may even be one of the subconscious reasons why they overeat. These are the kinds of people who are attracted to the "health spa" or "health club," a fast-growing and profitable phenomena of our times. Not since the era of the Roman Baths, has the health club service been quite so fashionable as it is right now. The ancient Italians enjoyed beautiful surroundings, efficient attendants, hot springs, cold plunges, and massage, and we have rediscovered these patrician pleasures in our own century.

The advertisements lure the public with soothing promises to make things better, no matter what the problem. "Overweight? Underweight, tense, bored?" International Health Spas invite you to get into shape in a two-week crash course which will cause you to "lose up to 15 pounds and inches in only 2 weeks." (That's if you're overweight, of course. If you're merely tense and bored, you'd better make that clear, so that you'll get into the appropriate program.)

The 10-Step Course includes (1) a complete figure or physique analysis, (2) individual instruction in the world's most modern gym, (3) relaxing Finnish sauna, (4) cleansing Turkish steam, (5 & 6) soothing whirlpool and refreshing swim, (7) decongestant inhalation room for that clear feeling, (8) Swedish massage, the frosting on the cake, for which you have to pay extra, (9) "top it off with a glowing bronze tan in *Tse Biam* tanning rooms," and (10) "a new you!" Naturally, if you read all the way through this ad, you have absorbed the international flavor of the venture and are ready to "make this your best summer yet" for only $24—limited offer with the advertisement. It's much cheaper than taking a trip abroad!

Another International Health Spas advertisement advises you to "take a second look—Clothes don't make the woman. She makes them! So if you have more or less than there should be, we've got the fastest and surest answer." Nevertheless, they seem to have slowed down, because this time you lose pounds and inches "in only 30 days while you enjoy the luxury of New England's most posh super spas." With this ad, the cost is $48, but then this program is for twice as much luxury and twice as long to enjoy it.

If you are intrigued by the exclusiveness of a posh spa, you may be interested to know that only three percent of the American public can find the leisure and the money to bask in the pleasures of the spa routine—despite the large showy advertisements in almost every major newspaper. Three percent doesn't sound like many, but it represents a large *number* of persons, and the figure is growing by leaps and bounds. This promises to be one of the healthiest business enterprises the future decade has to offer. For one thing, the price has at last come into the reach of the middle-class income, whereas previously only the very wealthy were able to afford this kind of total body worship.

There are, in our country, several *really* exclusive and expensive "Fat Farms" where upper-income ladies have been able to retire for two weeks for a "vacation" and come back to their usual round of activities revitalized and refreshed and refirmed for the social whirl. These ranches, or resorts, have been in existence for many years; now, finally, almost any person can afford a taste of the full beauty treatment the spa invites you to experience.

There isn't a thing that the spa can do for you, however, that you cannot do for yourself, except to provide you with the opportunity to use gym equipment that you might not have in your own playroom—and to offer you encouragement while you one-two-three your way to that proverbial "new you."

As far back as March, 1968, the magazine *Science News* printed a warning by the A.M.A. to weight reducers seeking moral support in the group therapy of a commercial health club. They stated then that it's of the utmost importance that a person who wants to lose weight have a physical examination by his doctor before participating in any of these programs. "Adequate treatment of obesity," the A.M.A. declared, "is often a more complex matter than diet and exercise, the usual club regimen. While simple overeating and under-exercising may be a cause of obesity, significant overweight frequently has a genetic, metabolic, or psychological component which requires medical diagnosis and treatment. Because there is no single cause of obesity, there is no single proper treatment to correct it."

This is good advice, and it might have been followed more faithfully by the public, especially by those who suffer from the "significant overweight" they mention, if there had been all along a warmer welcome and a more reliable treatment by the physicians whom the obese consulted. Instead, it seems that doctors were generally bored by the condition, except for those who intended to "specialize" in treating the obese with a dazzling and expensive array of pills.

The Massage Is the Message

Apparently, the "massage" aspect of certain health spas which cater exclusively to male clients is one of the newest interpretations of one of the oldest pastimes. The advertisements are usually smaller and may be recognized by the heading "For Men Only." One "Swedish Sauna Massage Parlor" offers their facilities to help you "unwind," plus a "Eucalyptus decongestant chamber to relieve colds or hay fever. Infra-red to relax nerves. Finnish Hot Rock Sauna to relieve the body of lactic poisons and excess fluid. Whirlpool with hot bubbling mineral water to relieve aches and nervous tension. Miami Sun Room with ultra-violet lighting for early tans. And refreshments in our bachelor lounge." This ad closes with the suggestion that you call "Sonya" for more details.

Meanwhile, Sonya appears in another ad for the same parlor with a slightly different emphasis: "Beautiful Young Goddesses will pamper you"—and one of the goddesses is pictured wearing nothing as far as the eye can see and evidently named "Breathless." "For discreet gentlemen . . . FEELING IS BELIEVING . . . Call Sonya . . . appointment not necessary."

This kind of Swedish Parlor is not to be confused with a regular co-ed kind of health spa that really intends to work on your physical fitness. Not long ago, several cities were the scenes of police raids on "massage parlors" that offered rather overt "forbidden pleasures . . . for men only" that went somewhat beyond stimulating massage. Things in the health field, as we see, can get out of hand.

But the question remains—is massage good for you or not? Properly administered by trained professionals in a soothing environment (no young goddesses this time!), it can be both stimulating and relaxing. It can also improve your circulation. Massage should be firm and brisk, but never to the point of seeming like punishment. When it is administered by someone who is not strong enough, it is ineffective. If given by an untrained or incompetent person, it will not only fail to achieve the benefits that are possible, but it may even do damage. However, it must be understood that even the best kind of massage by a well-trained person will not rid you of excess fat, nor will it correct or improve a physical disorder or disease. Enjoy massage—but don't expect it to reshape your body into one like that of the movie star you most admire.

"Tenting Tonight on the Old Camp Grounds"

There are health spas that don't entirely exclude some of the attributes of the posh health clubs, but their offerings are a great deal more modest. Into this category fall the diet camps which are directed mostly toward young people and children. Usually these camps don't make outlandish promises in their advertisements, but they do state that they will reduce weight in pleasant surroundings with "fun" for those who attend. Some have medical people (other than a regular camp nurse) and nutritionists on their staffs, while others describe themselves as "non-medical trim-down camps." This can be a good opportunity for a young person to participate in a structured exercise and sports program. Since this will be at some distance from the well-intentioned but often inhibiting advice of his parents, it could result in some real benefits for a person in the difficult teen years. It is particularly at this time of life that home-nagging seems to work at cross purposes with a youngster who is trying to help himself to reach a specific health goal through diet. Many doctors have found it much easier to work with a teenager on a diet when his parents did not comment or interfere in any way. Therefore, a camp can be an ideal way of starting on the right road, if the meals are carefully and sensibly planned.

Here, as in everything else, you have to "shop around" and find out which camps have a reputable history. With room and board included, such a program is not inexpensive. For your teen-ager to have a summer of fun-filled weight-reducing can easily cost around $1,500.

Trends in Getting Trim

It's one of the ironies of our era that the dangers of sedentary life have inspired business to solve the problem with all manner of automated devices designed to take the work and sweat out of exercising. There are, however, a couple of general precepts that you can keep in mind while trying to sort the wheat from the chaff. First, the greater the claims made for a new piece of exercise equipment, the more suspicious you should be. By this rule, the contrivance that claims to take off the most weight in the smallest amount of time is the least credible. Secondly, the more passive you are encouraged to be in using the machine, the less good it is liable to do for your health and fitness. The more active you have to be in using a device, the more actual exercise is being provided by it.

Considering the tenor of our times, it should come as no surprise that computers are now being pressed into service to solve the dilemma of our fat society—

and (here's the surprise) the new program, called Counterweight, is being sponsored by General Mills, who has also helped to promote all those cake mixes, each one a little moister and more fattening than the other. For a one-time fee of $78.00, a computer interprets your answers to a lengthy questionnaire about your eating and exercise habits.

If those of you who have personally experienced the fallibility of computers are a little discouraged by this development, you are urged to keep an open mind and remember that it takes time to get the bugs out. True, if the wrong hole gets punched, the computer may put you on a regimen of 100 finger bends a day or a diet of prime ribs of tadpole, but the goal of the program is to help the individual to lose weight within the framework of his own life style. For the atmosphere of authority, the 13-week program includes educational meetings held in a Minneapolis hospital.

As the year 2000 approaches, we hardly dare project what wonderful apparatuses will be placed at the disposal of the unfit with what fantastic promises of instant improvement. One could anticipate exercise by remote control, exercise in simulated outer-space weightlessness, exercise with the aid of atomic activators, and other amazing developments, with or without Richard Strauss' theme music. It is to be hoped that those who truly want to improve their physical fitness will hang on to some of the good things of the past, like walking, swimming, dancing, and bicycling down a pleasant country lane.

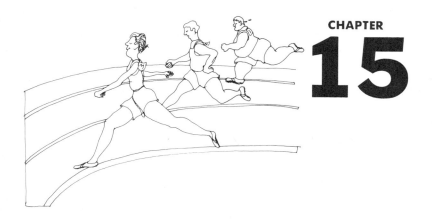

Exercise Has the Inside Track

There's more than one way to exercise a fat cat. Any man is bound to find it a thoroughly enjoyable experience to sit in his easy chair, sipping a cool beer, while Debbie Drake goes through a series of body stretches and deep-knee bends on his TV screen. For the women, there's Jack LaLanne flexing his muscles with a flashing smile. Anyone would find it much more relaxing, while cozily tucked in bed, to watch "Janaki" in place of the 11:00 p.m. news. And all of us can tune in to Maggie and the Beautiful Machine to see if any of our neighbors got on the show this week.

These voyeuristic exercises may be stimulating and entertaining ("Janaki" is especially sensuous and absolutely graceful), but they will do little for anyone who doesn't actually participate in the exercises. If you feel silly going through the motions with the voice on the TV supervising, the only part of you that will be getting exercised is your eyeballs, and the trouble with America today is there's too much eye exercise and not enough body work.

Strange, but true—Americans who don't exercise often believe they get enough exercise (through their daily activities), while those who *do* exercise are much more concerned about whether they're getting *enough* exercise to keep themselves physically fit. The May, 1973 Special Edition of the President's Council on Physical Fitness and Sports *Newsletter* offers some revealing statistics. About 49 million adult Americans "do not engage in physical activity for the purpose of exercise." That's 45 percent of the 109 million adult men and women! Half the total adult population (63 percent of American women and 38 percent of American men) have *never* participated in competitive sports— and that includes their school years! Four out of five Americans say they've never been advised by a doctor to exercise.

Those who do exercise choose their methods from a wide range of activities. Of these 60 million adults, six-and-a-half million jog, 14 million swim, another 14 million do calisthenics, and 18 million ride bicycles. By far the most popular form of exercise is walking. Nearly 44 million use this pleasant and inexpensive method. There's also weight lifting, of course, and various sports and games. Bowling is especially popular, as are golf, softball, tennis, volleyball, water skiing, and skiing.

Many adults who engage in these exercises and say they believe they're getting sufficient exercise actually don't do them often enough or long enough to benefit from them. One bike ride a week, jogging on Tuesdays and Saturdays, or taking a swim on Sundays —this is not really exercising for fitness. But many persons are confident that such slight routines constitute "enough exercise." The one exception is among the walkers. They seem to be a more conscientious and persistent group. More than half the adults (men and women) who walk for exercise, do so daily or almost every day, and three-fourths of them walk at least 20 minutes each time out.

If you're not really that "outdoorsy" and prefer exercising in private, there are other alternatives. Your office, while your boss is out to lunch, or your dressing room at home may be more to your liking as the arena of your progress toward fitness. In that case, isometrics (as opposed to isotonics, which require actual movement) may be what you've chosen to solve your fitness problems and suit your preferences.

Neat Exercises for Small Spaces

Isometrics, in case you haven't read a magazine for the past ten years, is a method of physical exercise in which one set of muscles is briefly tensed in opposition to another set of muscles or in opposition to a solid surface. It has the advantage of being a neat thing to do that requires no more space than you'll find in an ordinary clothes closet, if you really want to keep your physical fitness program a secret. There are kinds of isometric exercises that you can do while you're sitting at your desk in the office, and no one will notice the difference, unless they catch you gritting your teeth. Even driving the car, you can be tensing up your stomach muscles for a trimmer figure.

Remember the horror show of electrical devices for muscle stimulation? The electric devices use a technique of muscle contraction closely related to iso-metrics. Both cause the muscle to contract by building up tension without shortening or lengthening the ends of the muscle. Although isometrics have been effective in some ways, they have a built-in drawback, just like their electrical counterparts. By causing the muscle to contract in a particular position, the exercise becomes highly specific and is effective only in that position. There is no weight loss or reduction in size from con-tractions like that. Also, an isometric exercise will not improve flexibility. Flexibility requires movement so that stretching and contracting of muscles, tendons, and ligaments will occur.

What isometrics can do is firm up and tighten "lazy" muscles that make you look flabbier than you need to look. Although they won't make you smaller, isometrics will make you "neater."

Big Exercises for Wide, Open Spaces

Dr. Kenneth H. Cooper, author of *Aerobics,* is credited with having begun the national craze for jog-ging. Based on a point system of building up toward a goal of fitness, aerobics concentrates on exercise that increases the body's supply and use of oxygen. There's no hiding this exercise program in a closet, or even in your own backyard—aerobics means running, walk-ing, swimming, cycling, and other "breath-taking" ac-tivities.

Provided you're in good physical condition, these exercises are excellent ones when adapted to your age and stage of physical fitness. Dr. Cooper claims that his program will provide you with the following benefits: you'll breathe easier, because the muscles in your chest will be stronger (the program forces you to go a little further and faster each time you do your chosen exercise or activity); your heart will pump more efficiently; you'll increase the number and size of your blood vessels; you'll have more blood circulating . . . and better circulation; you may lower your blood pressure.

Dr. Cooper has, with the assistance of his wife, adapted this method of exercising to women, with a specially designed regimen suited to their special needs. A major in the United States Air Force, Dr. Cooper's original program was worked out with Air Force personnel and was necessarily male-oriented.

If you don't enjoy jogging and don't own a bicycle, you can still try Dr. Cooper's program, with something as uncomplicated as walking. The point is not what you do, but the way you do it. The idea is to exercise long enough to step-up your heart beat and oxygen in-take. More than an attempt to build up muscles, aerobics seeks to exercise your heart, lungs, and circulatory system.

Dr. Cooper encourages you to work up to your goal gradually, not to overdo, to dress appropriately, and to drink plenty of water to replace what you'll lose in perspiration. A medical check-up is advised for anyone over the age of thirty. *If you honestly adhere to these precautions,* aerobics can have a lot of benefits to offer anyone who wants to become more physically fit—or to help along a diet program with increased healthful exercise.

It's an interesting point for dieters that strenuous exercise before a meal actually depresses appetite. Dr. Cooper explains that one may not feel very hungry at the particular time of day when the exercise is performed, because the activity shunts the blood away from the stomach, decreasing the desire for food.

Graceful Exercises for Mirrored Rooms

If you can't quite imagine yourself "jogging in place" in front of a mirror—all that flesh bouncing around!—and you're not the type to flex your biceps at odd moments of the day, there is another alternative, a graceful, slow-moving system of exercise designed to increase your mental tranquility while it promotes your health. It's called *Tai Chi* (pronounced tie-jee), and it's been practiced widely in China since the T'ang Dynasty, 618 to 907 A.D. Edward Maisel, a Harvard and Princeton-trained rehabilitation expert who was once the Research Director for the New York Institute for the Crippled and Disabled, has written a comprehensive guide to this exercise system called *Tai Chi for Health.*

Tai Chi originates from the Chinese theory of opposites—Yin and Yang. As Mr. Maisel explains it, "The words 'Tai Chi' in Chinese mean this whole circle made up of the Yin and the Yang, and the movements of *Tai Chi* supposedly follow these principles. Throughout the exercise, opposites succeed each other in the progression of movement. Thus the hand which is above descends, and the hand which is down comes up. The leg which bears the weight (the strong, or Yang leg) becomes empty and weightless as the weight shifts to the other leg. The arms continually describe circles, large or small. The hands move through globe-holding positions—in theory, the hands are holding the Yin-Yang circle. No movement is complete in itself: it is always becoming something else, moving toward its opposite. And the end of every movement or gesture is not an end but the beginning of another movement."

There are 108 movements in all making up the *Tai Chi* routine, made up of 37 basic actions. The rule of thumb, says Mr. Maisel, is that if it doesn't feel "light and natural," it is wrong. Mr. Maisel also stresses that age is no barrier: "Old persons are as capable of this slow-moving exercise as the young; the refreshment produced by the soothing movements is, if anything, more exhilarating to them."

If time to exercise is your problem, and you find that the only moments you have free are just before retiring, *Tai Chi* could be an ideal choice. According to Mr. Maisel, it calms and settles your nerves as it drives away an "anxious, worried, nervous, tense, or excited state of mind." Doesn't that sound relaxing? And the best part is, it really is an exercise that will help to keep you in good shape as much as many others. For this system, you'll really need Mr. Maisel's book as a guide to the complex and intricate movements of *Tai Chi*—and try a little soothing music to accompany your Yin-Yang mood!

Rolling through Those Rolling Hills

Want to be a crises solver? There *is* a way that you and others like you could bring a great improvement to the nation's physical unfitness, the pollution problem, the energy crisis, the traffic snarl, and even the parking problem—by joining the growing ranks of bicyclists!

In countries where gasoline is scarce or very expensive and automobiles are out of the reach of most of the population because of their low incomes, people have turned, of necessity, to bicycles for everyday transportation. In Red China today, for instance, most people go through their daily activities by either bicycling or walking, getting healthful exercise because no alternatives are available. Alternatives are plentiful in the United States, but many of our current problems have caused us to take another look at and give a new evaluation to the bicycle.

Designed as a pleasant excursion vehicle, mostly for children or tourists in resort areas like Nantucket where bike-trails run alongside the motor roads, the bicycle is now being reconsidered as a sensible relief alternate to the congested commuter conditions on our highways and in our cities. And there's the added benefit to the pedaling commuter in the vigorous and stimulating exercise that this form of transportation provides. Rather than "robbing Peter to pay Paul," this kind of solution is more like paying Paul to benefit Peter as well.

At present, there is evidence of serious proposals and actions to encourage the increased use of bicycles. Some states are already making available a small percentage of highway funds for the construction of bike trails (and, bless them, hike trails, too!). The so-called "Bike Lobby" in Oregon succeeded in interesting enough Oregon citizens to impress their state representatives, who voted for and passed House Bill 1700, which directs that one percent of the state's Highway Fund be set aside to establish a system of bike trails and footpaths wherever a highway or even a street is being constructed or modified. Areas such as abandoned rights-of-way lend themselves beautifully to such use, and one such right-of-way near Portland, Oregon, is already being converted into a bike-and-hike trail.

Good ideas sometimes catch on—the neighboring state of Washington has allocated one half of one percent of highway funds for the same purpose. But in California, Governor Reagan vetoed a measure that would have put $60,000 a month into bike trails because it "wasn't right" to use money meant for automobiles and mass transit systems on a bike-and-hike system. Logic might lead one to conclude that roads are designed to get people from point A to point B, their tax money pays for these roads, and any effective mode of transportation, including walking and biking, justifies utilization of that money.

California Senator Alan Cranston's Bicycle Transportation Act (S. 2440) may succeed in "creating bike paths for the whole country," including California. With this bill in effect, cities and counties would be able to tap the Highway Trust Fund to build separate roads for bicyclists. New Jersey, Michigan, Missouri, Kansas, New York, and Ohio are also considering bills of their own.

Compare the uncomplicated bicycle with the demanding automobile on which we've come to rely so heavily. The automobile causes more deaths yearly than diabetes and arteriosclerosis combined, and it is the leading cause of air pollution—the nitrogen, oxides, lead, hydrocarbons, and other poisons it spews into the atmosphere, and the resulting ozone and photochemical smog assault every inch of our bodies, from our eyes to our red blood cells. University of Southern California's Dr. Oscar J. Balchum recently demonstrated that the ozone resulting from automobile engine pollution actually disintegrates the walls of many red blood cells, in a process which is chemically similar to what happens when butter turns rancid.

Of course, automobiles are necessary to cover distances too long for biking, but one way you can improve your fitness and the environment also, is to use a bike for commuting to nearby stores and work locations. This will encourage the government to build more bike trails, which will make cycling that much more pleasant. Things could escalate this way along a much pleasanter path than the creep-and-beep highways we suffer through now.

Keep Moving—and You'll Keep Young

There's no question about the fact that America is youth-oriented, almost to the point of worshipping the early years of life. This is easy enough to observe through the slant of most advertising—grandparents are expected to be slim and vigorous, wives are encouraged to dye their hair so that their husbands will love them more, and no one is permitted to feel sluggish on the day of the Big Fair, without having a friend recommend a good laxative. Television fare does not tax the mature intellect, nor are movies with titles like *Widget Meets the Werewolves* produced with the tastes of sophisticated older people in mind. Mini-skirts and flared trousers were not designed for the usual middle-aged figure. To anyone over the age of thirty, this may begin to appear like a large-scale plot.

While many of the assets of maturity are overlooked by the present culture, which is a deplorable state of affairs, the emphasis on having a youthful figure is a healthful one. And it is *body activity* that will restore a youthful figure and reduce appetite at the same time.

Authorities at the University of Illinois' Department of Physical Education got some interesting results in an experiment with five overweight non-exercising men, ages 35 to 46 years, who volunteered for an exercise program in running. Without their following a specific diet, there was a decrease in body fat and an increase in the ability of the men to perform during the course of the program. Their walking and jogging (alternately) became progressively more vigorous, and the time and distance covered in each session increased considerably by the end of the 16-week program.

The key here is that it was body *fat* that decreased. As we get older, it is the increased fat that accounts for most of the weight gained, as the researchers, Drs. Lawrence B. Oscai and Ben T. Williams point out. "Fat-free weight remains unchanged or decreases slightly with advancing years." Their conclusion: that exercise *can* help to rid the body of excess fat.

Exercise has not always enjoyed a good reputation among the weight conscious. There are a number of discouraging statistics which inform you that it would take 36 hours of walking to take off one pound of overweight or that it takes seven hours of walking to burn up the calories you get from a hamburger. Actually, this is not quite the way it works in real life, especially if you take the long view (which is the one we recommend). Walking an extra half hour a day will take off five pounds a year. And walking is a very mild exercise. If you were to add an hour of tennis, swimming, or bicycling to your daily activity, eating the same amount of food as always, the loss could go up to 25 pounds of excess weight in a year's time.

There is a popular misconception that exercise is not effective in weight loss because it stimulates the appetite in direct proportion to the increased activity. On the contrary, according to Dr. Jean Mayer, while appetite follows activity in the range of normal activity in animals, sedentary animals (those most likely to be obese) actually show a *loss of appetite* with an increase of up to one hour of daily exercise. This same principle applies to humans. Exercise that helps to get rid of body fat always means effort on your part, not reliance on passive methods, or techniques buttressed by shiny chrome equipment and luxurious surroundings.

Keep your body moving, and it will stay younger than you believed possible. Non-use is the greatest enemy of "the beautiful machine." On the other hand, if you haven't been doing much more than turning the key in your car's ignition and a few TV knobs for the past ten years, go at it slowly and build up your strength. Stay within the bounds of common sense (for this, after all, is supposed to be the *reward* of maturity) and allow a gradual progression to greater exertion. Activity should be vigorous enough to bring up your body heat, but not enough to exhaust you. Select something pleasant that will work in well with your normal routines. For instance, you could park your car a half hour away from your usual destinations and walk the rest of the distance, on a daily basis. Remember that exercise is best when it involves the whole body, not just parts of it that you want to slim down. Find sports you enjoy, get involved, and participate three or four times a week (more, if you can).

Keep your body moving, moving, moving, because that's where life and youth will be found—in healthful activity!

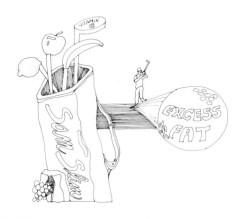

16

It's a Whole New Game

At this point, we've learned some things about fad diets, reducing aids, effortless exercise gadgets, health spas, cult programs, pill therapy, surgery, and other currently popular methods of weight control. They're either expensive or they don't produce long-term results or they're dangerous—or all three of these may be true!

With fad diets, for example, you probably will lose weight initially, but, as soon as you quit the diet, you'll put those pounds right back on! Many people own two wardrobes just to keep up with these rapid changes. Improper dieting may have further encumbered you with physiological disorders and emotional frustrations. Drastic by-pass surgery for the truly desperate may succeed in slimming the obese, but it is always terribly uncomfortable, and it can be fatal. You can be vibrated at home with your exercise machines or massaged down at the local health club—it feels good, but it doesn't do anything miraculous for your figure. It's no wonder that people get discouraged and decide to chuck the whole business! (If an individual has been on the weigh-in see-saw, losing then regaining a number of pounds, he *would* be better off to stay fat—it is less of a strain on the heart!)

Despite the agonized bravado of those who cry "fat is beautiful," however, obesity is not a happy nor a healthy condition with which to live. Carrying an extra 25 pounds of weight is about as much fun as being sentenced to haul around a 25-pound sack of potatoes for life. And it isn't really necessary to sentence yourself to this handicap. Common sense is the key, and the rules of good health are the formula. You can re-educate yourself to a new life-style that really will give you long-term results in weight reduction— it won't be fast, but it will be sure!

One of the most important factors in beginning this new life will be to approach it in an affirmative manner. If you believe in a negative way that you are punishing yourself by adopting a healthful regimen, the program is almost automatically doomed to failure. The same is true, in a more subtle sense, of a program which you think of as temporary. Why should it be temporary, if it's good for you? Temporary regimens are just to be endured, to be gotten through as quickly as possible so that you can get back to normal eating patterns (Those same eating patterns that got you into so much trouble in the first place)—if you think in this fashion, your new life is in jeopardy again.

Instead, it is necessary to believe that you are entering a way of life that will be permanent, which will allow you to discover new ways to satisfy your hunger while keeping your body fit with healthful exercise. There is no reason why this would not be thoroughly enjoyable *in the process.* Shakespeare said, "There is nothing either good or bad, but thinking makes it so." A healthful life style, logically, must be more enjoyable than any other, because good health is the basis of all other pleasure.

The seven steps with which we propose to accomplish this new life style are not complicated or difficult to understand at all. They are all steps which you can take by yourself; they do not require an outlay of huge sums of money, the chore of constant visits to the doctor, or the dependence upon group meetings. Once you decide you really want to do something about your weight, you can get started right away (and it's very important to *get started!*)

You won't run into any difficult obstacles. We offer no magic formulas, no fantastic instant results, and no effortless miraculous change. It will take some time to achieve your goal, but this will give your body time to adjust to your changing figure, and you will avoid subjecting it to a fast unhealthy shift. The unsightly sagging skin that often accompanies crash dieting won't be one of the problems with which you'll have to contend. The beauty of it (and of you!) will be that the weight you take off in this manner *will stay off for the rest of your life,* as long as you continue to follow the simple precepts of a healthful diet. Your life will probably be longer, and it certainly will be happier!

Instead of thinking in terms of "dieting" and "losing weight," think of physical fitness as a way of life. You can change and improve your body. Healthy helpings of optimism, faith in yourself, good common sense, and the determination to enjoy life while keeping fit will head you along the right road—straight toward your goal. You don't want another interim program but a permanent change of life style. In a family environment, the individual needs of the members can be accommodated and woven into the fabric of this new life. Not only will all the family benefit by leading healthier and more vigorous lives, but the attitudes and harmony engendered can continue on to bless future generations.

Survival in the Supermarket

The importance of *good food* cannot be emphasized enough! If you are in a position to grow your own vegetables and fruits, naturally and organically, you are lucky and to be envied. Many persons, however, are forced to depend on outside sources, and, therefore, we urge you to seek out the most healthful food supplies that you can find. Mass production and mass merchandising through supermarkets has increased the variety and the quantity of foods from which we may choose, but there are attendant evils. You, the buyer, must be aware and beware. It is the quality of foods that has suffered in our society.

We're not encouraging anyone to work up a good case of paranoia on the subject—we are, however, suggesting that you be very canny and knowledgeable when you wheel that supermarket cart blithely down the brightly-lit aisles. Learn all you can about consumer abuses, about the psychology of advertising, and, most of all, about nutrition. You'll need all the armor you can muster to face the motivational "up" music wafting through the store and still come out a winner in food value.

Nutrition is not only a survival measure. It's a complex system of supplying the body with nourishment that will provide the energy necessary for your body to fulfill its function requirements, provide repair and replacement of body structures worn out by work and play, and provide the *means* by which the body utilizes the nutrients that accomplish all this. (Some nutrients help other nutrients to work at their fullest capacity.)

There are five main food elements to consider:

Carbohydrates are the starches and sugars, the most immediately accessible form of energy. Starches are mostly found in cereal products and some vegetables and fruits. The sugar in food is usually *sucrose;* another important sugar, *lactose,* is found in milk.

Fats, made up of fatty acids and glycerol, provide a sense of satiety and are another source of energy. "Visible" fats include oils, butter, margarine, and shortening added to food. "Invisible" fats are fats already present in food, like the fats in meats, fish, eggs, the butterfat in milk, et cetera. Some fatty acids are "saturated;" others are "unsaturated." Too many saturated fats in the diet can raise the cholesterol level, which may, in turn, invite physiological problems.

Protein is especially necessary for growth and the maintenance of body structures. Protein is also another source of energy—more extended energy than carbo-hydrates provide. The highest quality protein is found in meat, fish, eggs, milk, and cheese; however, some protein is present in all natural foods.

Vitamins cannot be manufactured by the body; you must depend on the food you eat or on vitamin supplements to supply them. Vitamin A, found in green and yellow vegetables, fish liver, and fish liver oils, is necessary for the welfare of your skin and bones. The B vitamins are primarily active in manufacturing the health of the nervous system. They also help your system to utilize the sugars and starches you eat. Good sources of the B-complex are organ meats and unrefined cereal grains. Ascorbic acid, vitamin C, is essential for the maintenance of all body tissue; it prevents scurvy and acts to secure the body against infection. This vitamin is found in citrus and other fruits, and in most vegetables, particularly potatoes. Vitamin D is necessary for the body's utilization of calcium. It is available from fish, eggs, liver, liver oils, milk, butter, and also obtained from sunlight on the skin. Vitamin E is required for circulatory health. It appears in most fresh seeds and nuts, in unprocessed vegetable oils, and is especially concentrated in wheat germ. Vitamin F, unsaturated fatty acids, specifically linolenic acid, linoleic acid and arachidonic acid, is required for prevention of fatty deposits which can lead to circulatory disorders (most prevalent among natural grains, fruits, vegetables, nuts, separated vegetable oils, fish liver oils, and seeds). Vitamin K protects against hemorrhaging and may help to prevent spontaneous abortions. It also protects against some cancer-producing substances. Alfalfa, spinach, kale, carrot tops, and all green leafy vegetables contain vitamin K. The bioflavonoids, sometimes called rutin or, vitamin P, prevent hemorrhaging, lessen stroke possibility in high blood pressure cases, and protect against the harmful effects of x-ray. Green peppers, citrus fruits (in the white membrane that you lose when you squeeze them for juice), grapes, prunes, plums, black currants, and rose hips are good sources. When used in conjunction with vitamin C, both vitamins become more effective.

Minerals are essential for growth and the maintenance of body structures, too, although they are sometimes overlooked. Calcium, magnesium, and phosphorus are essential parts of bones and teeth, and calcium is also important to blood clotting. Iron is a vital part of hemoglobin—the red coloring matter in the blood. Minerals also assist in maintaining the composition of digestive juices and the fluids in and around body cells. Other vital minerals include iodine, potassium, sodium, sulfur, zinc, cobalt, manganese, and copper. Your body requires differing amounts of these several minerals— ranging from large amounts (calcium and phosphorus, for example) to very small amounts or "traces" (iodine, and copper, to name a few).

Water must not be forgotten in discussing the body's needs, but frequently it "goes without saying." By water, we don't mean coffee, tea, coke, soup, or any other liquid. Every day's intake ought to include several glasses of pure, plain water, which plays such a vital role in health. Its importance might be underlined by remembering that you can live longer without food than you can without water—so it ought not to be neglected and ignored.

This, admittedly, has been a rather whirlwind tour of nutritional needs. If you've already read a lot about nutrition, you may feel you know all that you need to know, in which case, it's only a matter of keeping all this in mind when you shop and cook. If, on the other hand, you feel you're lacking in essential knowledge in this whole field, hopefully you will study one of the many excellent books on this vital subject for in-depth coverage. Once you're really conversant on nutritional needs, the most complicated part of your healthful new way of life will be accomplished.

But, there you are, still in the supermarket, wondering what to buy. Lean meats, liver, fresh fish, chicken, fresh vegetables of all kinds, fruits, eggs, cheese, butter, and whole-grain products that haven't had all their nourishment squeezed out of them. Unsalted nuts and unsaturated oils more or less complete the picture of what your shopping cart should contain. As a consolation (in case you're having a twinge of deprivation) take a good long look at the folks whose carts are bulging with whoopie pies, six-packs of cola, hot dogs, potato sticks, and washed-out frozen dinners. These food buyers will not be the pink-cheeked, energetic, slim type you're aiming to be on your new food plan. Your food budget will not suffer from avoiding junk foods—and you'll be spending your money for real, beautiful fruits and vegetables instead of cardboard containers with *pictures* of real food on them and very little by way of nutritional value inside.

So, be strong—arrive at the store with a list (*after* you've eaten), learn to rely on fresh, seasonal foods, and don't for a minute talk yourself into some non-food with that good, old excuse—"it's the family favorite!" The family will develop *new* favorites, if given the opportunity.

How To Say "Good Morning"—and Mean It!

The first step in any healthful reducing plan is to take a good look at your breakfast—what there is of it! If you're like most Americans, you "haven't time for anything more than a glass of orange juice and a cup of coffee," or you "just can't digest a lot of heavy food first thing in the morning," or you "always have a good big bowlful of frosted vitamin flakes." If this is true of *your* morning habits, this is the very first place to begin to re-organize your daily food plan—and it's a *must!*

Breakfast is the most important meal of the day, especially to reducers. The energy provided at breakfast is what you use to sail into the day's activities and coast past the pastry temptations of the morning. If you move vigorously and tend to a number of errands by walking rather than "letting your fingers do the walking" by phoning, you will, of course, burn up more food energy, thus contributing to fat loss. But, if all you have in your stomach is a glass of fruit juice and some coffee, chances are you will be drooping on the vine by 9:30 a.m., and your stomach will be rumbling with hunger. Nor will an ounce of something "shot from guns" be any more substantial. Either way, you'll be ready to grab a sugar doughnut or a Danish because you "need the energy."

First of all, think of what the word *break-fast* really means. You've actually been fasting through your night's sleep, and your body is ready for some nourishment. It will not be fooled for long by a cup of sugared coffee. That's why your morning meal should contain some protein food. Scrambled eggs (add a sprinkle of wheat germ!), cheese melted on whole-grain toast, chicken livers, or a small sandwich steak will provide you with this essential food element. You'll find your own favorites, once you get the idea. Granted, you'll have to get up about twenty minutes earlier than usual, but a good breakfast can go a long way toward helping you to enjoy mornings more.

Also important is some kind of fruit in the morning—and remember that it doesn't have to be citrus. In spring, strawberries are an especially good choice for reducers; in summer, consider melons, particularly cantaloupe. Make a list of fruits according to their carbohydrate content, putting the ones with the lowest content at the top. Choose whole fruits rather than juices, fruits that are in season rather than those that are not, and consult your list to determine which fruit of the present season is the best for reducing. It will be the one nearest the top of the list. Fruit will provide you with natural sugar, with needed vitamins, and will aid in digestion.

Try not to rely on bread, but, if it seems absolutely necessary with your eggs, choose a whole-grain variety, and have half a slice (or a very thin whole slice).

Farm-fresh eggs are much tastier and better for you than supermarket-storage eggs. A little butter is permissible, because fat contributes to a feeling of satiety and helps to mobilize your body's stored fat as well—polyunsaturated fats, however, are preferable.

If you eat this kind of breakfast every morning (not just on weekends), your blood sugar will remain high for a much longer period of time during the day, and you won't suffer from an intense craving for a jelly doughnut about 10:00 a.m. More than that, you also won't be as tempted to raid the refrigerator late in the evening! This is because your whole body will be on a proper schedule of energy and will feel nourished by this excellent start to your day—and the other good foods you will be choosing for later meals.

High-Test Fuel for a First Class Engine

Step Two is to determine to make the protein foods a central part of *every* meal, and to play down the role of carbohydrates in your menu plan. No necessary food element should be cut entirely from your regimen, however, and that includes carbohydrates. While it is true that carbohydrate is a fat-producer in fat people, it is also true that it is not safe to depend upon an unbalanced diet. We suggest, therefore, that you cut out the kind of carbohydrate foods that have no real food value in favor of healthful carbohydrate foods, such as fruits and vegetables, to a reasonable proportion of the day's fare.

With vegetables, you can make a list, just as you did with fruits, with the foods containing the least carbohydrate at the top. Again, choose foods in season, and don't avoid the yellow vegetables entirely, just because they are richer in carbohydrate than most of the green ones. What you can do is to make the starchier vegetables the ones of which you only have one helping (that's about a half cup) while you fill up on the less starchy ones, the vegetables at the top of the list. You'll find many leafy green vegetables are good choices, and, if you have lots of these in salads, often, you'll be doing two good things for yourself.

Raw foods are much richer in vitamins than cooked ones, and the polyunsaturated oils that we recommend for salad dressings contribute to your day's fat allowance and promote satiety. There's a side benefit, too: salads take a lot of *time* to eat and provide plenty of *chewing*. A salad for lunch, with eggs or cheese, will keep your mouth busy through a whole lunch hour, while your friends with the sandwiches will be finished in ten minutes. With all that munching, you'll have no reason to feel deprived!

Your vital protein allotment should be taken in lean, unsalted meats. Eggs, fish, unsalted nuts, and cheese are also good choices. Beware of ham, luncheon meats such as salami, hot dogs, bacon, and other salted meats, because salt will cause you to retain fluid and make it more difficult for you to lose weight. Since women tend to have a problem with water retention at the beginning of their reducing plans anyway, there is no use in compounding the difficulty with excess salt.

You'll find that a concentration on the protein foods will carry you through the day's activities with a feeling of well-being, with plenty of energy to move around more, and without hunger pangs. Protein foods have a staying power that no other food can match, so don't ever be tempted to eat *less* by skipping this important fuel.

How To Avoid That "Empty Feeling"

By "empty feeling," we're not talking about hunger. You'll be avoiding hunger with a concentration on protein foods. We mean that emptiness which results from eating too many "empty foods"—foods which contribute only bulk to your body, without any real nourishment value. Individuals who rely upon these empty meals will find themselves lacking in energy, in good looks, in stamina, and many other qualities which we all desire.

This leads us directly to Step Three. For many persons, this is the hardest step, although it's not a difficult one, unless you eat in restaurants every day.

It's easy enough to recognize the emptiness of soft drinks and candy, but there are other foods that were once healthful and wholesome which have been done in by modern processing. These are not as commonly recognized.

Products made of refined flour (whether it's bleached or unbleached) are empty foods. All the good nutrition of the wheat germ has been milled out by the so-called improving process of making them white. Adding synthetic nutrients to make up the deficit is not equal to what nature provided in the first place. Therefore, they have nothing to contribute to your reducing plan but a lot of carbohydrate that you don't need. Avoid them. Substitute other good foods instead.

Whatever grain products you eat should be made from natural whole grains so that they will be a useful component of your meals. Wheat germ is probably your best cereal source of nutrients, and it can be used in so many good ways! Sprinkle it on salads, on fruit or eggs; add it to meat loaf instead of breadcrumbs—you'll enjoy the delicious "toasty" flavor. If you're hooked on bread, limit yourself to two slices per day, and make certain that it has been made of unrefined, naturally-grown wheat grain.

It's a good idea, too, to give up salt (or cut down drastically). As we have mentioned before, salt retains fluid in your body and makes it more difficult to lose weight. Soy sauce and MSG cause the same problem, with the added worry that you may be allergic to MSG —some people are, and it makes them ill.

We are not, however, suggesting that you resign yourself to flavorless food—far from it! In fact, we don't want you to feel resigned to anything, because that's such a negative feeling. What we suggest is that you readjust your thinking and use more imagination in seasoning your meals. Garlic and onion are wonderfully flavorable in many dishes. Herbs are good additions and so are many spices.

Here's just a beginner's list of flavoring for experimentation: oregano or basil (or both) on anything that has tomato in it; nutmeg on squash; ginger on carrots; basil on green beans; lots of fresh parsley and chive on potatoes; dill on salads (or ground anise, or basil); rub beef with a cut garlic clove, paprika on pot roast or in stew, thyme and sage for chicken dishes, lemon with veal or fish (also good on most vegetables); wheat germ, chive, or basil are excellent on eggs. The possibilities are limitless, and you'll find more and more emphasis on using herbs in cooking in the latest cookbooks. Many people are even growing their own herbs to use in cooking, and nothing could be more delicious.

You should never *need* to add salt to your foods, because food in its natural state contains enough salt to meet your body's ordinary needs. The taste for salt is an acquired one, and it can be "de-acquired." After about two weeks without salt (and *with* other flavorings) you probably won't even miss it. Your palate adjusts and enables you to enjoy the really good, natural tastes of food. The first thing you'll notice is that many foods, especially vegetables, seem *sweeter* once you have given up salt.

Speaking of natural sweetness, whatever need your body has for sugar can be best supplied by the natural sugars in fruits and vegetables rather than the much-advertised refined sugar products. Candy, cakes, pies, and cookies are almost pure carbohydrate, with all of the adverse effects carbohydrate has on the obese metabolism and none of the food value offered by fruits and vegetables.

The chief ploy of sugar-product advertisers is that sugar gives you a fast "boost in energy." It is true that sugar raises your blood sugar for a time, but it soon plunges far below what it was in the first place, leaving you feeling worse than you did, more listless, more tired.

In 1968, government statistics revealed that the so-called average American consumed 96 pounds of sugar per year! This poor John Doe is to be pitied. His body was so busy burning up the 96 pounds of sugar that much of the rest of the food he ate was stored as fat. He probably gained weight, and, chances are, he spent many hours at the dentist having those sugar-coated teeth repaired.

Some researchers seriously question whether sugar

is the chief source of energy for muscles. In 1954, Dr. Ruben Andres of Johns Hopkins University reported that his development of a technique to measure substances carried to and from muscle led him to conclude: "Muscle, like other tissues of the body, meets its energy requirements by degrading certain substances. In the course of this degradation, oxygen is consumed by the muscle. It has generally been held that most of the oxygen consumption of muscle occurred during the process of degrading sugars, and that these sugars are the major energy sources of the muscle. The present investigations are interpreted to suggest that the older idea is not true, and that sugars may not be the major energy for muscle."

Dr. William M. Fowler told the Ninth National Conference on Medical Aspects of Sports that "There is no evidence . . . that sugar as a pre-event supplement increases athletic performance."

M.I.T. nutritionist Warren M. Navia told the American Chemical Society in September 1967 that sugar has been refined to such a degree that it is devoid of the vitamins and minerals essential for its metabolism.

Dr. Norman Jolliffe, in his book *Clinical Nutrition,* showed that protein foods actually contribute more to the body's energy requirement than empty foods like sugar or sugar-based products.

Sugar has also been linked to heart disease. Dr. John Yudkin of the University of London reported that patients with myocardial infarction consumed more sugar than normal persons. Dr. Clifford Anderson, a California doctor, warned people to "take a close look at the sugar bowl if they intend to avoid heart attacks." He declared that sugar builds up fatty tissues on the inside of coronary arteries which could clot and cause a heart attack.

The "quick energy" that sugar seems to give the body comes from a rush of glucose into your bloodstream, a rush of insulin to metabolize it, and a subsequent depletion of sugar in your blood. Beatrice Trum Hunter, in her book *Consumer Beware,* points out that "Excessive amounts of sugar consumed for 'quick energy' are burned at the expense of inadequate amounts of protein and fat which supply essential elements necessary for proper metabolism."

For sustained energy, depend on high protein foods and natural carbohydrates found in fruits and vegetables. This enables your tissues to store glycogen and to release it as glucose to your blood in a controlled, steady, long-lasting manner. (The best thing for you would be to get rid of your sugar bowl entirely, or use it for something decorative—a small bouquet . . . or a goldfish!)

Eating sugar products *depresses* energy in the long run because it reduces the ability of the body to oxidize glucose, the process by which energy is generated. It is inaccurate of "experts" to casually group all carbohydrates together. They don't all behave the same way. Various forms of carbohydrates differ in how they are metabolized. The December, 1970 issue of *Nutrition and Metabolism* included a study by Drs. A. E. Bender and Pushba V. Thadani, of Queen Elizabeth College in England, which clearly demonstrated a definite difference in the metabolic pathways traveled by the various form of carbohydrates.

Let's use the example of a car engine to better

understand how energy is produced in the body. When you burn fuel in your car engine, you get heat, which is converted to energy. When you burn glucose in your body cells, you are performing the same process—far more efficiently. When oxygen combines with glucose, it oxidizes or burns the glucose and creates heat and energy. The by-product of this combustion is carbon dioxide which you expel when you exhale.

Regardless of the source, your body converts about 68 percent of all the food you eat into glucose for conversion into energy. The other 32 percent is used for building and repairing the body. Not only sugars and starches, but also fats and proteins can be changed by the body's mechanism into the kind of sugar that the body needs to produce energy.

What the Bender-Thadani tests have shown is that *the ability of the body to oxidize glucose is reduced if the source of the glucose is sucrose, which is refined sugar.*

Dr. John Yudkin, in his book, *Getting the Most Out of Food,* explained that one of the nutritional disadvantages from a high consumption of sugar is that "it leads to disease." Besides the well-known matter of tooth decay, Dr. Yudkin cites "stomach ulcers, diabetes, and, above all, coronary thrombosis."

Step Three, then, is a radical step—it requires you to give up refined sugar and its products, refined flour and its products, and salt, other than what is naturally present in foods. This will provide you with a healthier diet and a chance to reduce your weight at the same time, reduce it in such a way that it will never be regained. These changes in your food selection are meant to be permanent, and they will help you to keep the weight you lose off permanently.

We can't leave it there without telling you how this can be accomplished with the least trauma to your tummy! The important word here is substitution. When you cut out salt, you add or substitute spices and herbs and other natural flavoring agents. When you eliminate refined sugar, and all the desserts made with it, you substitute fresh fruit desserts made with the same loving care you used to lavish on cake frosting. (Fresh fruit and cheese is a dessert with real continental style, anyway, and you can be proud to serve it anytime.) Natural honey or unsalted nuts may be used on this food plan, also. When you stop buying refined flour and its products, you substitute whole grain foods instead. The purpose here is two-fold: to provide you with a balanced diet and to prevent you from feeling deprived, so the substitution technique is an important one in making lasting changes in your life style.

More Bounce to the Ounce

Step Four suggests the intelligent selection of natural food supplements to supply the vitamins, minerals, and enzymes that are lacking in processed foods and further destroyed by cooking. It is especially important to feel and look well while you are taking off weight, and this step will insure your enjoying optimum good health with lots of energy to spare for Step Seven (we're getting to that!)

Be certain to include the whole range of B vitamins in your natural food supplements plan—these vitamins are important to the metabolism of carbohydrates; they're the flame that ignites the fuel. But the B vitamins are team workers, and should be taken with other vitamins and minerals.

By taking food supplements (natural supplements are best), you can be certain that what has been lost in "civilizing" foods (packaging, storing, soaking, steaming for hours, tenderizing, re-coloring, and the like) will not be lost to your body's needs.

Divide and Conquer

Many persons, when they decide to diet, courageously give up meals. Some even make it a practice to eat only "one good meal a day." Such a fine example of misplaced courage probably hasn't been seen since General Custer rode bravely out into the prairie.

Instead of giving up meals, what we suggest you do, in Step Five, is to *eat more meals*. (Remember . . . we didn't say *more food*.) Try dividing your food allotment into smaller portions—six smaller meals a day will help to prevent hunger and make it easier to lose weight—rather than three stuffing meals. You'll feel better because your body will be utilizing the food you eat more efficiently. It will be consumed to keep you supplied with energy, because there won't be enough left over to store as fat. (It's a little like keeping your bills paid up to date rather than combining them into one big fat deficit.)

Experiments have shown repeatedly that the level of fats in the bloodstream rises in persons who eat only one or two heavy meals a day for their daily fuel. Studies completed in 1961 and 1964 demonstrated that the serum lipid level in patients declined when their meal portions were simply made smaller and given more often. This means the likelihood of their experiencing hunger was much less, and it can work that way for you, too.

Psychologically, it's a good idea if one of your meals during the day is still a real "dinner," whenever you are accustomed to having that meal. Again, you avoid the feeling of being deprived. But your new dinner should be a great deal lighter than the full starchy fiasco that most people in our society consume.

Another reason for making one of your meals "dinner" is that there are certain vegetables that most people will never eat as a snack—have you ever seen someone go to the refrigerator and take out a half cup of turnip or a couple of stalks of broccoli? These vegetables are very good for you and are also, most naturally, a component of what is called dinner.

And dinner is a charming family or social occasion that is good for you emotionally. Since it's important to be happy while you're getting healthy, we don't want you to neglect anything that contributes to your emotional welfare.

With this in mind, we suggest you rearrange your meals into six much smaller, lighter ones, including a dinner.

Munching to Your Heart's Content

You'll like Step Six! Following the logic of Step Five, it becomes okay to munch your way through a few snacks during the day, but you will have to be highly selective about what foods you consume. No more pretzels, potato chips, candy bars, or soggy little pies. Instead, choose raw vegetables, toasted soybeans, raisins, seeds, unsalted nuts, and fruit. Not only will you be satisfying your snacking desire, but you'll be getting minerals, vitamins, and enzymes. While helping yourself to these goodies, you'll be helping your body as well.

The Lively Way of Life

Step Seven means exercise, move around and burn up the food you eat every day. With all that good nutrition, you'll be feeling like a little extra activity anyway!

Some people actually become alarmed at the thought of exercise. They envision a home gym fully equipped with expensive push-and-pull gadgets, or hours of backbreaking calisthenics, or sprints across town. Not only is it unnecessary to go to such extremes, it can actually be dangerous to embark on a punishing exercise routine after leading a sedentary life for years. Here, too, as in every other step, let common sense be your guide.

Start slowly, with easier forms of exercise, and build up your ability and strength cautiously—but doggedly. You'll be able to tell when you can advance the pace and amount of your activities. Remember not to push yourself to exhaustion ever!

Whatever activities you choose, the best ones involve the whole body as much as possible, and they require real effort on your part. It's important not only for weight control but for health itself to keep your body toned up and flexible. Exercise helps to delay the effects of the aging process magnificently!

It is really necessary to the reducing plan presented here that you get more exercise than you have been getting in the past, so don't neglect this important step. Whatever you decide to do, do it at least four or five times a week, and, in-between times, get outdoors and enjoy a brisk walk! Sitting around the house just makes you feel like eating more; moving around and being active makes you think less about eating. As your energy output increases, so does the burning of food intake. You don't eat more when you exercise; you just enjoy it more!

Just one of the many side-benefits of exercise—although you may feel tired physically after a workout, you'll find that worries and mental fatigues will be lessened. Many persons feel mentally as well as physically invigorated by exercise!

Now, let's recapitulate the seven steps: *One*—Start the day off right with a good breakfast, and that means a protein breakfast. Depend on protein rather than caffeine to see you through the morning. *Two*—Design *all* your meals around a protein food as the main attraction. Rely on the "protein hold" rather than the "carbohydrate jump." Monitor your carbohydrate foods, and, remember—"Carbohydrate weighs; protein stays." *Three*—and that's three foods to ignore from now on . . . refined flour products, refined sugar products, and salt. Substitute something else instead. *Four*—Insure against vitamin, mineral, and enzyme deficiencies by taking natural food supplements that will replace the nutrients lost in processing and in cooking. *Five*—Eat smaller meals oftener, rather than bigger meals three times a day. But have a "dinner." *Six*—Snack on real foods like seeds, raisins, soybeans, fresh raw vegetables, and fruits. *Seven*—Get more exercise; make some total body activity part of your everyday routine. Don't overdo, but do help burn up your food intake in this pleasurable way.

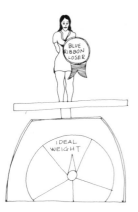

CHAPTER 17

The Winner Loses— the Loser Wins

You may be saying to yourself, "What a peculiar program this is! My interest is in losing weight, and no where in these seven steps are diets or calories or scales mentioned!" That's just the point! "Diets" don't work. The inevitable failure outcome is built into them, because they are designed to be temporary measures. We've avoided words that have come to mean something negative and punishing, in favor of offering you a way to a more healthful, vigorous life—and weight reduction, too!

The important thing is to think in a positive way about physical fitness. Calorie allotments you find in books are generalized and unrealistic. You are *you,* unique, and like no one else, and your reducing plan has to be designed for your particular needs. Of course, you'll eat less, exercise more, and feel better for it! You'll weigh yourself once in a while to see how you're doing, and you'll look in the mirror often. (Don't weigh yourself more than once a week—but be sure to weigh yourself at least once a month.) Most important, getting over a heavy reliance on empty, fattening foods and moving around more will surely take weight off and keep it off.

Treat Yourself Royally

There's something to be said for dining, rather than wolfing down a snack at the kitchen sink. A nicely set table, attractive food, good linen, and pleasant company all contribute to the feeling of having eaten a meal that was satisfying. As we have already seen, external stimuli mean a great deal especially to the obese. So, treat yourself royally, make a fuss over your meals, eat slowly, and enjoy every bite. If you're not dining alone, try a little conversation between bites. Serve dinner in courses; the longer it takes, the better.

Just one word of warning: never put serving dishes on the table so that you can help yourself to more. Bring to the table exactly what you propose to eat. If you have to serve "family style," because there you are surrounded by your family, all of whom can have extra helpings, make up your mind that what you put on your plate the first time around is all you're going to have.

If there's a tablespoon of food left over, either in a serving dish, a pan, or on a child's plate, don't eat it. Save it or throw it out. Put it away, but not in your stomach. It's better to waste food than to be unhealthy and unattractive. If you have a dog, you probably know you're *not* doing him any favor by feeding him a left-over spoonful of mashed potatoes. Treat yourself as well as you would a pet.

Party It Up

By all means, go to parties while you are slimming down. They're good for the morale, and what's good for the morale makes it easier to lose weight. Party food is notoriously fattening, but there will probably be some things which you can enjoy nibbling. Platters of raw vegetables are "in" currently, and, if this is served, you can help yourself with abandon. Avoid olives (too salty) and the kinds of oily, salted nuts that are often set around in bowls at parties. Any kind of cheese you have to cut is okay, but don't have crackers, chips, or dips. Avoid luncheon meats, ham, and cocktail franks. Mushrooms (if not stuffed with bread) and chopped chicken liver are not only delicious, but they won't ruin your figure either.

Most important, if you over-indulge due to the fact that the hostess prepared a fattening snack which you've never been able to resist and she stood by while urging you to try it, don't spend three days mourning the failure of your "plan" (while eating things you shouldn't because "it's no use anyway"). Go right back to your usual healthful meals starting the very next morning and no great damage will have been done. The real damage would be to give up.

We don't recommend drinking, but, if the spirit of the occasion calls for it, try to drink dry wine or dry vermouth. Avoid liquor, beer, and sweet wines (like sherry or port).

Husband Keeping

While it is human nature to overlook the obvious, it is difficult to understand why women will ignore the health danger that obesity represents to their families, although they may be very much aware of the responsibilities of housekeeping. Let's assume that the woman is the chief cook in the home; attractive and good-tasting meals are important, but so are health and nutrition. By the same token, although it's important to the comfort of the family that the home be clean and cozy, it is also important to the family that each member of it enjoys the benefits of feeling fit and energetic. An overweight husband needs the attention of carefully prepared meals designed to trim him down while keeping him in good spirits, just as an obese child does.

Remember, it is better for the morale of the obese member of the family if everyone eats the same foods, more or less (meaning a little less for the chubby one). It is also a lot easier for the cook. The foods which are healthy for the dieter are also good for everyone else, so no one will be deprived. The dieter may have to stick to one helping of certain foods, but, in the main, everyone can enjoy the same meals.

The family shopper will be surprised at how much is saved by not buying potato chips, crackers, pastries, cokes, and similar snack foods. Splurge with the savings on a little more fruit, fresh vegetables, mushrooms, cheese, fish, and meat.

An overweight husband or chubby child are usually the first ones to be found rummaging through the refrigerator for a snack between meals. Obviously, if you have "forgotten" to buy chocolate-covered ice cream or marshmallow cakes, no one will be able to fill up on those. A hungry person will eat a ripe fruit or a celery stick or a piece of cheese instead, if those things appear in attractive array in the refrigerator.

A few hard-boiled eggs are a good thing to have around, as are unsalted nuts, grapes, and melon. Carrot sticks and radishes look pretty and taste good without ruining the figure. Cottage cheese seasoned with chopped celery leaves and dill or chive is an inviting high-protein snack for the "midnight raider." Fixing these foods and keeping them in the refrigerator takes less time than making a cake, even with a "mix."

If you are a woman reading this book, take a realistic look at your family. Maybe *you'd* like to take off ten pounds once and for all, but is there someone else you love who needs to lose weight even more? A lot of men in our society die in their fifties while their widows live twenty lonely years longer. In the long run, husband-keeping is more important than housekeeping and more deserving of a lot of careful, loving attention.

Burning Your Bridges

As you lose weight, you find, of course, that those bulky sweatshirts you've been wearing to hide the bulges are now hanging from your shoulders. Slacks are threatening to fall off with every step. It definitely becomes time to buy a new wardrobe. No one is going to notice that you've lost weight as long as you're still slouching around in old army fatigues or caftans.

This is a beautiful moment for the formerly-fat to savor, one of the new rewards of success to replace the old reward for failure, which was food and more food. It is also a time when you can really be daring. *Give away all your old clothes* immediately, lest you remember that you have another wardrobe waiting for you should you back-slide. Instead, make up your mind that you will never endanger your health or your new wardrobe by regaining the weight you have lost.

How can you be sure? The knowledge that you will have nothing to wear but a barrel if you gain over five pounds will go a long way toward inspiring you to weigh yourself at least once a month which is what you should do. A gain of over five pounds is a real hazard, and one of the main reasons why is that it tends to make you feel hopeless and helpless; that kind of thinking drives you right back to the satisfactions you used to find in fattening foods.

While you're at it, there's a few other things you can give away, like cookie jars, cracker tins, and cake plates. Buy a fancy fruit bowl, instead. You can't give away your refrigerator, but you can keep it filled with good foods that won't make you fat, and snacks that are delicious but not starchy. Remember, what you don't buy, you can't eat. And, just to be sure you won't be tempted by the lure of the shiny jars and brightly-colored boxes that the supermarket displays so invitingly, don't ever go shopping on an empty stomach. You'd be surprised what willpower you can develop when your tummy is full.

There's no need, however, for you to start a worldwide crusade. When in Rome, or Grand Rapids, or Oshkosh, by all means eat the native food, but eat it *selectively.* The same applies to visits to your parents' home or to the homes of unenlightened friends. It isn't one day's digression that will make you fat again; it's what you eat day after day in your own home that counts.

Life without an Adding Machine

With the life style we propose, you aren't going to notice any instant, dramatic results (other than a feeling of new energy and well-being due to eating a real breakfast and getting enough of every kind of nutritional element during the day). You're not going to take off "seven pounds in seven days" or "25 pounds the first month." Our way is slower—but it lasts a lot longer!

Steadily, but certainly, your body will move towards its proper balance. It will get back in tune, you will feel less tired and more motivated to lead a full, active life. Your figure will change to what it should be for your body type, but it will do it in a way that gives your system a chance to keep up with the disappearance of those extra pounds. You'll avoid the haggard look and sagging skin that accompanies fast, unhealthy weight loss, not to mention the snappish temper that results from semi-starvation. All of this, because you won't feel "starved" during the process, and you won't be hungry.

There will be plenty of good-tasting foods on which you can fill up, yet you will avoid the uncomfortable feelings that often result from the flashy, zero-carbohydrate diets. You will monitor your carbohydrate intake with your fruit and vegetable lists, but you won't be involved in the higher mathematics of counting every calorie or gram you consume.

You'll get to the point where you'll eat only as

much as your body needs. You'll even avoid the transition from reducing regimen to maintenance regimen (the point at which many "dieters" begin to replace what they've starved to lose) because you won't be thinking in those terms any more. Once out of your childhood years, you *know* when you're overeating. If your appestat doesn't tell you, your intellect does.

"It's Not Nice To Fool Mother Nature"

The "negative" reducing approaches that this book has explored demonstrate their failures far more often than any accidental and incidental successes they may occasionally achieve. The body (and the mind) resist punishment and abuse but respond readily to sensible and sensitive treatment.

A high-protein style of eating can be expensive, but it needn't be. You can choose the less expensive high-protein foods—it doesn't have to be prime rib! Also, if you balance what it does cost you against the cost of fraudulent reducing "aids" and devices, against expensive group meetings and resort health programs, against costly medical and hospital bills brought on by obesity-promoted diseases and disorders, you will have to agree that the program we suggest is a real bargain —not just financially either!

Welcome to a New World

The goal we envision is within reach of all of us. A physically fit society is a strong, active society— a viable society. By enjoying fitness and normal weight, we will be eating better, living longer, and experiencing life in a more exciting way. We will pass these benefits on to future generations through example and teaching.

Despite all the past failures you may have experienced, you can really look forward to a wonderful new world of good health and proper weight—you can help yourself by following the few general rules this book proposes—and you *can* change your weight permanently to the right weight for *you!*

Happy living! Why should you settle for less?

Index

A

aerobics, 233-235
alcoholic beverages, choice of, 269
American Society of Bariatrics, 92
amphetamines, effects of, 162, 163, 183
  production of, 183, 184
  types of, list of, 165
  use of, 184-186
anxiety, appetite and, 20
appestat, role of, 15, 17, 18
appetite, depression of, drugs for, 162
  exercise and, 241
  function of, 18-21
  influences on, 19, 20
  regulation of, experiments with, 17
    influences on, 19
    obesity and, 21
appetite distractors, central-stimulating, 162
appetite suppressors, effectiveness of, 191-196
  side effects of, 193

B

"Bacon and Eggnog Diet," 116
bariatrics, 91, 92
basal metabolic rate, stimulants of, 163
bath additives, 199
belts, as reducing aid, 198
Benne Method, as body shaper, 207, 208
beverages, choice of, 269
bicycling, as exercise, 236-239
biofeedback, 158-160
blood, circulation of, sauna treatments and, 213, 214
blood pressure, weight and, 41
body shaping, courses for, 202-205
  effects of, 205, 206
body types, classification of, 29, 30

body wraps, 204-208. See also *body shaping*.
boredom, appetite and, 20
brain waves, types of, 159
breakfast, need for, 251-253
bulk producers, 164
  list of, 166
bust, developers for, 201, 202

C

caffeine, products containing, 149
  use of, 149
    effects of, 150
calisthenics, as exercise, 39
calorie(s), absorption of, heredity and, 34, 35
  consumption of, sexual activity and, 39
    social controls on, 77
calorie charts, 132-136
camps, for dieting, 227, 228
cancer, saccharin and, 148
carbohydrates, as food element, 247
  dieting and, 48
  fat formation and, 99
  role of, 143
cellulite, 199-201
chewing, weight loss and, 110
chewing gum, dieting and, 148
  digestion and, 149
children, obese, diabetes and, 81
  hyperinsulin and, 81
  parental influence on, 82
  peer attitude toward, 80
  obesity-prone, feeding of, 79
  overweight, numbers of, 80
coffee, as dieting aid, 149
  use of, effects of, 149-151
computers, diet programs and, 228, 229
culture, obesity and, 87
cyclamates, 148

D

deaths, diet pills and, 171, 172
    drug-related, 181, 182
    obesity and, 74
dehydration, sauna treatments and,
        211
diabetes, obesity and, 25
diet(s), duration of, 75, 76
    fad, types of, 113-145
    formula, 119-121
    influences on, 43
    list of, 124-129
    types of, 113-145. See also
        name of diet.
diet camps, 227, 228
diet clubs, 92. See also name of
        club.
diet drugs, appetite and, 19
    deaths from, 171, 172
    role of, evaluation of, 186-196
    side-effects of, 19
dieters, numbers of, 76
dieting, carbohydrates and, 48
    clubs for, 92. See also name
        of club.
    computerized, 228-229
    cost of, 274
    statistics on, 75, 76
digestion, chewing gum and, 148
digitalis, use of, 175, 176
diuretics, effects of, 164, 165, 169
    list of, 166
    use of, for water-retention
        problem, 26
Dr. Atkins' Diet Revolution, 138-
        139
    reactions to, 141-143
drug therapy, 161-196
drugs, appetite and, 19
    control of, 170
    deaths from, 171, 172, 181,
        182
    diet. See *diet drugs.*
    interaction of, 179-182

E

eating, external cues in, 52
    frequency of, 262, 263
    speed of, effects of, 58
    types of, effects of, 63
eating habits, hypnosis and, 62
ectomorph, description of, 29
emotions, appetite and, 20, 64, 65
    hunger and, 48
endomorph, description of, 30
energy, sugar and, 259
environment, diet and, 43
    obesity and, 27
excitement, appetite and, 20
exercise, appetite and, 241
    as reducing aid, 230-242, 264,
        265
    benefits of, 239-242
    isometric, 232, 233
    muscle tone and, 38, 99
    obesity and, 37
    types of, 232-239
Exercise Sandals, 221, 222

F

fad diets, types of, 113-145
family, food planning and, 270,
        271
fashion, as motivational factor, 31
    obese person and, 88
fasting, 130-132
    as treatment, 97-99
    long-term, complications of,
        132
fat, as food element, 247
    formation of, 98, 99
fat cells, increase in, 32
"Fat Farms," 224
Fat Mobilizing Hormone (FMH),
        139
fat non-obesity, 32
flavorings, choice of, 256
Fletcherism, 110
fluorine, tea and, 152

food(s), as emotional substitute, 50
  elements of, 247-250
  "empty," 255
  party, choice of, 269
  preservatives in, 152-153
  symbolism of, 64
  types of, choice of, 252-264
food planning, family considerations in, 271
food supplements, in daily diet, 261, 262
formula diets, 119-121
frustration, appetite and, 20

G

genetics, obesity and, 24, 26-28
glucose, as energy source, 260
  defective metabolism of, 25
gluttony, 61
grains, as nutrient source, 255

H

HCG, effectiveness of, 189-191
  use of, 173-175
Health Mattresses, 221
heart attacks, obesity and, 43
heart disease, obesity and, 40, 41
  sugar and, 258
heat stroke, sauna treatments and, 212
herbs, choice of, 256
heredity, calorie absorption and, 34, 35
  obesity and, 25-36, 42
hormones, use of, 173-175
human chorionic gonadotrophin. See HCG.
hunger, recognition of, 52
  tension and, 45
hyperinsulinism, 25
hypertension, obesity and, 41
hypnosis, eating habits and, 62
hypometabolism, 41

hypothalamus, appestat and, 15
hypothermy, effect of, 205, 206

J

"Jet-Start Diet," 115
jogging, as exercise, 233-235
juveniles, obesity in, 79-83. See also children.

K

ketosis, carbohydrates and, 139

L

lactose, as food element, 247
lean tissues, fat formation and, 98

M

machines, as reducing aids, 215-222
massage, 225-227
  benefits of, 226
Mattresses, "Health," 221
"Mayo Egg Diet," 117
meals, frequency of, 262, 263
men, average weight of, 76
mesomorph, description of, 29
metabolism, definition of, 21
  rate of, manipulation of, 21, 22
  stimulants of, 163
  thyroid pill and, 22
Metrecal, 119
milk, skimmed. See skim milk.
minerals, as food element, 249
morphology, of obese persons, 28-32
muscle(s), stimulation of, devices for, 218, 219
muscle tone, exercise and, 38, 99
  stimulation and, 219

N

National Association to Aid Fat
   Americans (NAAFA),
   role of, 56, 92, 93
"night eating," 59
nutrients, types of, 247-250
nutrition, influence of, on appetite, 20

O

obesity, as social problem, 78
   as status symbol, 86
   culture and, 87
   cures for, fraudulent, 100-103
   death and, 74
   definition of, 6, 23, 98
   degree of, determination of, 8
   diabetes and, 25
   diagnosis of, 8, 9
   effects of, 40-42
   genetic factors in, 26-28
   heredity and, 42
   "home tests" for, 8
   in juveniles, 79-83. See also
      children, obese.
   in underdeveloped countries,
      11
   inherited, 24-35
      likelihood of, 26-28
   long-term, 70
   old remedies for, 105-111
   prognosis for, 57, 70
   psychological factors in, 46
   types of, 32, 33
   walking and, 37
overeaters, types of, 67, 68
overeating, causes of, 51-54, 61
   control of, drugs for, 162-165
   emotional factors in, 47
   obesity and, 9, 10
overweight, definition of, 6, 7

P

party foods, choice of, 269

pep pills, 183-186
personality, of overeaters, 67
pharmacotherapy, use of, 161
pills, diet. See diet drugs.
   "pep," 183-186
   "rainbow," 176-182
   reducing, contents of, 169,
      170. See also diet drugs.
preservatives, in meats, effects of,
   152-153
protein, as food element, 247, 248
   deficiency of, disorders caused
      by, 137, 138
   need for, 253
   sources of, 254
psychological factors, appetite and,
   20
   obesity and, 46
purgatives, effects of, 164, 165
   list of, 166

R

"rainbow pills," 176-182
reducing aids, drugs as, 165
   fraudulent, 100-103
   types of, 167-170
reducing equipment, 197-229
Regimen, 122
Relaxacizor, 216-218
rice diet, 113, 114, 118
"Rockefeller Diet," 136

S

saccharin, cancer and, 148
salt, in daily diet, 256, 257
saunas, 208-215
   blood circulation and, 213,
      214
schizophrenia, treatment of, fast-
      ing and, 131
"secret eating," 59
sedatives, effects of, 164
   list of, 166
self-deception, 7

self-image, 54-58
sexual activity, calorie consumption and, 39
skim milk, food value of, 147
    production of, 146
snacks, between-meal, choice of, 263
spas, 222-225
spices, choice of, 256
spot reducers, 220
starch, as food element, 247
starvation, therapeutic, 130-132
starvation diets, as treatment, 98
status symbol, obesity as, 86
steam baths, effects of, 213
stimulants, metabolic, 163
sucrose, as food element, 247
sugar, as food element, 247
    energy and, 259
    heart disease and, 258
    use of, 257-260
sunstroke, sauna treatments and, 212

T

Tai Chi, as exercise, 235, 236
tannic acid, tea and, 151
taste, acquired, 48
tea, as dieting aid, 149
    use of, effects of, 151
tension, hunger and, 45
thin obesity, 32
thyroid extract, use of, 173
thyroid gland, role of, 22
thyroid pill, metabolism rate and, 22

thyroxin, role of, 22
tissues, lean, fat formation and, 98
TOPS, 91
tranquilizers, effects of, 164
    list of, 166

V

vegetables, choice of, 253
vitamins, as food element, 248

W

walking, as exercise, 37
water, as food element, 249
    weight loss and, 211
water retention, as symptom, 25
weight, average, 76
    blood pressure and, 41
    excessive, effects of, 40-42
    loss of, chewing and, 110
    proper, maintenance of, 33
        271-274
Weight Control, 156-158
weight charts, 7
Weight Watchers, 91
wheat germ, as nutrient source, 255
will power, role of, 9, 10
women, average weight of, 76
work capacity, 37

Z

Zen Macrobiotic Diet, 153-156